Dealing with PTSD and Trauma

CRAFTED BY SKRIUWER

TABLE OF CONTENTS

CHAPTER 1: UNDERSTANDING PTSD

- Defining PTSD and its causes
- Recognizing common signs and symptoms
- Addressing key misunderstandings

CHAPTER 2: TYPES OF TRAUMA

- Different forms of traumatic events
- Why each event can affect people in unique ways
- Understanding single-incident vs. repeated trauma

CHAPTER 3: SIGNS AND SYMPTOMS

- Early indicators of distress
- Emotional and physical warning signals
- Knowing when professional support is needed

CHAPTER 4: HOW TRAUMA AFFECTS THE BODY

- The body's alarm response to danger
- Long-term physical impacts of ongoing stress
- Why acknowledging bodily reactions is crucial

CHAPTER 5: FINDING PROFESSIONAL HELP

- Different types of mental health professionals
- Approaches to therapy and medication
- Overcoming barriers to accessing support

CHAPTER 6: STRESS MANAGEMENT METHODS

- Breathing and relaxation techniques
- Mindful strategies for everyday tension
- Practical tips to reduce anxiety at home or work

CHAPTER 14: HELPING OTHERS UNDERSTAND

- *Sharing your experience safely*
- *Educating friends and family about triggers*
- *Setting boundaries around private details*

CHAPTER 15: OVERCOMING AVOIDANCE

- *Why avoidance feels safe but harms growth*
- *Approaches to facing what you fear*
- *Building a freer, less restricted life*

CHAPTER 16: EVERYDAY STRATEGIES FOR HEALING

- *Integrating coping into daily routines*
- *Sustaining positive habits over time*
- *Strengthening emotional resilience*

CHAPTER 17: HANDLING SETBACKS

- *Why setbacks are normal and not a failure*
- *Early signs and quick interventions*
- *Regaining your balance after a rough patch*

CHAPTER 18: REBUILDING TRUST AND BONDS

- *Healing relationships hurt by trauma*
- *Setting boundaries and improving communication*
- *Growing closer while safeguarding your well-being*

CHAPTER 19: KEEPING PROBLEMS FROM RETURNING

- *Relapse prevention and long-term self-care*
- *Adapting coping skills as life changes*
- *Maintaining a stable foundation for wellness*

CHAPTER 20: LOOKING AHEAD WITH HOPE

- *Embracing gradual progress and future goals*
- *Balancing acceptance with optimism*
- *Building a life shaped by resilience, not by trauma alone*

Chapter 1: Understanding PTSD

Post-Traumatic Stress Disorder (PTSD) is a mental health condition that can happen after someone goes through a very scary, harmful, or shocking event. These events might place a person in danger or make them witness something that deeply upsets them. Many people might think that PTSD only happens to soldiers who come back from war, but it can happen to anyone. A person might get PTSD after a car accident, a natural disaster like a hurricane or earthquake, a physical attack, or anything else that makes them feel extreme fear or distress. It is not a weakness, and it does not mean the person did something wrong.

Some people who go through very stressful or hurtful events might feel better after a while. Their sad or frightened feelings might fade on their own. But others might keep having strong distress that does not go away with time. They might have bad dreams, flashbacks, or feel stuck in the painful event. These reactions can last for many weeks, months, or years. When these feelings do not go away, it could be PTSD.

Below, we will look at how PTSD happens, some of the common reasons behind it, and why it affects different people in different ways.

What Is Trauma?
Trauma refers to a very upsetting experience that causes a lot of stress. Trauma can make a person feel shocked, frightened, or helpless. When this event is over, the body and mind might keep reacting as if the danger is still there. Trauma can come from many sources, such as violence, accidents, or personal loss. While some people recover faster, others need more time or help to feel safe and calm again.

If trauma keeps weighing on a person's mind, they can get stuck in a pattern of distressing memories and feelings. For some folks, these feelings fade when life becomes calmer. For others, the body and mind hold on to the pain. When this pain lasts and starts making daily life harder, it can lead to PTSD. Understanding what trauma is and how it acts on the mind and body is a first step to understanding PTSD.

How PTSD Starts

There is not one single reason why some people get PTSD and others do not. Many things can be part of the problem, such as the person's genetic makeup, how the body and brain respond to stress, and the type of support they have around them. When someone goes through a very upsetting event, their body goes into a high-alert mode to handle danger. This is often called the "fight, flight, or freeze" response. In healthy situations, once the danger is gone, the body slows down and returns to a normal state.

However, with PTSD, the body's danger response does not go away so easily. The memory of what happened can make a person feel as though the threat is still real, even if it is over. Nightmares, flashbacks, and strong reactions can keep happening because the mind is trying to make sense of the event. This mental struggle can make a person feel upset long after the event ended.

Common Symptoms of PTSD

People with PTSD can have many different signs of trouble. Not everyone will have the same kinds of feelings or thoughts, but there are some patterns that often show up:

1. **Re-experiencing symptoms**: These can include vivid memories, bad dreams, and flashbacks. During a flashback, a person might feel as if they are reliving the event. Their heart might beat fast, or they might feel sweaty or shaky. These re-experiencing symptoms can make a person feel like they are never safe.
2. **Avoidance symptoms**: A person with PTSD might stay away from places or things that remind them of the bad event. For example, if they had a car accident, they might avoid driving or even riding in a car. They might also try to push away thoughts, feelings, or discussions about what happened.
3. **Arousal and reactivity symptoms**: This might look like being jumpy, always looking around for danger, having trouble sleeping, or feeling easily annoyed. The person's body might be on edge, ready to act as if danger is around every corner.
4. **Changes in mood and thinking**: A person with PTSD might feel down, guilty, or alone. They might lose interest in things they once liked. They might also have strong negative thoughts about themselves or the world.

Not everyone has all these signs, and they can be milder or more intense from person to person. It is also normal for these feelings to come and go in waves. Sometimes the person might feel almost normal, and then something might happen that stirs up all the fear or sadness again.

Who Can Get PTSD?

Anyone can get PTSD if they go through or see something deeply upsetting. This includes children, teens, and adults of any age. Many people think only soldiers or rescue workers can develop PTSD, but that is not true. People who live through dangerous weather events, violent crime, or painful personal experiences can also develop PTSD. Even witnessing an event that happens to someone else can cause PTSD.

Children can get PTSD, too. They might act out or cling to adults. They might have trouble sleeping or wet the bed. They might feel scared and not know how to talk about it. Teens can also get PTSD, though their signs might look more like anger, mood changes, and pulling away from friends. Being aware that anyone can get PTSD helps us understand why we need to learn more about it.

Misunderstandings About PTSD

Sometimes people think that those with PTSD are "weak" or cannot handle stress. This is not correct. PTSD does not show weakness. It simply means that the person's brain and body are holding on to the stress in a way that is tough to shake off. Another misunderstanding is that PTSD always shows up right after the event. While many people do notice signs right away, it can also take a while before symptoms become clear. Some folks might seem fine at first, only to have signs of PTSD pop up months later when the stress or memory returns in some way.

Other times, people might think that PTSD is permanent or cannot be helped. This is not true either. With the right support, many people manage their PTSD, feel better, and regain control over their lives. Proper care might include counseling, medication, and learning ways to handle stress. Support from friends and family can also help.

PTSD and the Brain

PTSD has a lot to do with how the brain handles fear and stress. There are parts of the brain that are in charge of storing memories, handling emotions, and deciding what is safe or dangerous. One of these parts is the amygdala, which works like an alarm system for the body. When we face danger, the amygdala starts the body's "fight, flight, or freeze" response. Another important part is the hippocampus, which helps store and retrieve memories. With PTSD, the amygdala might stay on high alert for no real reason, and the hippocampus might mix up how it stores the traumatic memory, making it pop up in harsh ways.

It can be reassuring to know that the brain has a certain plasticity, which means it can adjust and change. Even if there are changes from trauma, the brain can learn healthier ways to respond. Counseling or therapy can help a person reprocess how they think about the painful event, while certain medicines might help manage the body's stress reaction. It is a process that might take time, but knowing the brain can change is a hopeful sign for many people.

Emotional Effects of PTSD

The emotional toll of PTSD can be big. A person with PTSD may feel fear, anger, shame, or sadness. They might blame themselves for what happened, even if it was not their fault. They might feel lonely if they think no one else understands. These strong feelings can make it hard to keep relationships going, stay focused at work or school, and find reasons to be hopeful.

It can help to remember that these emotional troubles are not signs of personal failure. Instead, they are natural responses to a harsh experience. Recognizing that these feelings are normal can allow the person to see that help is possible. The emotional weight might be heavy, but with help and healthy methods, it can lighten over time.

Behavioral Effects of PTSD

The stress of PTSD can push people to act in ways that others might not understand. They might suddenly become very angry at small things. They might avoid going places or seeing people they used to enjoy. They might feel numb, as if they cannot experience happiness or closeness. Some might begin to use alcohol or other substances to try to numb the pain. Sadly, these behaviors can create more problems in work, school, and relationships.

It is important to see that these behaviors are often attempts to handle overwhelming feelings. Recognizing the reasons behind them is the first step in getting better. With the right help, it becomes possible to replace harmful behaviors with safer ways to cope.

PTSD vs. Normal Stress

Feeling stress after a hard time is normal. Not everyone who lives through trauma will get PTSD. Some stress reactions might be short-lived. When the difficult event fades into the past, the mind and body often relax. But PTSD is different. It is not just stress. It is a lasting issue that keeps interrupting daily life.

One main difference is how long the troubles last and how intense they are. If a person cannot sleep for weeks, has repeated flashbacks, or avoids many activities because of fear, it might be more than just regular stress. A counselor or therapist can help figure this out and suggest next steps.

Why Early Help Matters

Getting help early can make a difference. If someone has been through a painful event and notices that they are feeling too anxious, jumpy, or sad to go about normal tasks, it is wise to reach out. Early help might mean talking to a professional who can suggest exercises for stress, or a doctor who can explain treatment choices.

Early help does not mean a person is weak. It is often the strongest step they can take. It is a way to keep things from getting worse and to learn skills to manage stress before it grows. In many cases, reaching out sooner can lead to quicker relief.

PTSD and Daily Life

PTSD can affect work, school, home life, and fun activities. A person might have trouble keeping their mind on tasks if they are worried or tired from lack of sleep. They might be nervous around groups of people. Even simple tasks like going to the store might feel too scary if there are triggers that set off painful memories. Over time, these changes can lead to isolation and shame.

Despite these problems, it is important to know that life can improve. Understanding the nature of PTSD is a strong foundation. It lets a person realize why they are feeling the way they do. Awareness also helps friends and family offer real understanding and support.

How to Know If You Might Have PTSD
Only a health professional can make a diagnosis, but you can ask yourself some questions if you suspect PTSD:

1. **Do I have intrusive memories or nightmares that make me feel as if the event is happening again?**
2. **Do I avoid people, places, or activities that remind me of what happened, even if it makes my life harder?**
3. **Do I feel on edge or jumpy most of the time, always watching for danger?**
4. **Have my moods or thoughts about myself changed in a negative way since the event?**

If the answer to some of these questions is yes, and these problems last more than a month, it might be time to talk to a mental health professional. Remember, seeking help is wise, not shameful.

Looking at the Bigger Picture
PTSD exists in a wide area of mental health concerns. It might appear along with anxiety, depression, or other stress-related problems. Sometimes people with PTSD do not realize that their anger, worry, or sadness might be connected to past events. They might think something is just "wrong" with them. By learning how PTSD works, a person can take steps to help themselves or a loved one.

Reasons to Learn About PTSD

1. **Better understanding**: When we know how PTSD works, we can make sense of the symptoms and not feel as confused or hopeless.
2. **Breaking down myths**: Knowledge helps end false ideas, like the thought that PTSD is only for soldiers or that it means a person is broken.

3. **Finding correct help**: The more someone knows about PTSD, the better they can talk to professionals, pick the right support, and learn helpful strategies.
4. **Providing support**: If a family member or friend has PTSD, knowing about it can help us be caring and patient.

Being Kind to Yourself

People who have gone through a harsh event can feel shame, anger, or guilt. They might think they should "get over it." But PTSD is not something a person can just forget on command. It helps to be kind to yourself. Remind yourself that your responses are normal reactions to something very difficult. This kindness can reduce the extra stress that comes from judging yourself or others.

Conclusion of Chapter 1

In this chapter, we looked at what PTSD is and how it can show up in daily life. We saw that PTSD can happen to anyone who faces a painful or dangerous event. The signs can be serious and long-lasting, but it is also clear that help is possible. Learning about PTSD is the first big step toward managing it.

As we move forward, we will explore different areas that relate to trauma, the various kinds of trauma that people can face, ways to cope with triggers, and methods to find safe connections. Being informed helps lay the groundwork for real change. With steady care, understanding, and support, people can learn ways to feel more in control of their mind and body.

Chapter 2: Types of Trauma

There are many kinds of events that can lead to trauma. It is not only big disasters like earthquakes or fires that harm a person. Trauma can arise from smaller, but still distressing, events that shake a person's sense of safety. Different events can lead to different problems, but they all share the potential to overwhelm the mind and body. In this chapter, we will look at several common types of trauma. We will also see why each type might affect someone in a unique way.

---

1. Physical Trauma

Physical trauma is harm to the body from accidents, violence, or other events. A car accident can be an example. If someone is in a bad crash, they might fear getting in a car afterward. The body might also hold on to the feeling of the crash, so even a small brake noise can cause panic. Other forms of physical trauma might come from fights, attacks, or any event that causes injuries to the body. Sometimes, repeated physical harm in a household can lead to ongoing trauma, where the person feels trapped and unsafe at all times.

People with physical trauma often need not only medical treatment but also support for their mind. The memory of pain or the image of what happened can keep returning. Some may blame themselves, thinking they did not act correctly or protect themselves enough. This can add a layer of guilt that stays long after the body heals. Physical trauma can be very serious because it can mix both physical and emotional pain.

---

2. Emotional and Psychological Trauma

Not all trauma involves clear physical harm. Emotional or psychological trauma can happen if a person experiences extreme fear, shame, or helplessness. This might come from bullying, verbal attacks, manipulation, or ongoing stress in the home or community. Sometimes, repeated harsh words or actions can leave a deeper scar than any physical injury. Emotional trauma can also come from witnessing violence or living under constant threat.

In many cases, emotional trauma is invisible. There might be no cuts or bruises to show for it. Yet, the person can be deeply hurt inside. They might have trouble trusting others or feel worthless because of what was said to them. They might relive hurtful conversations in their head and struggle to sleep. People often overlook emotional trauma, but it can be just as strong as physical trauma.

---

3. Sexual Trauma

Sexual trauma can be one of the most harmful forms of trauma. It includes any unwanted sexual act, threat, or pressure that leads someone to feel violated or forced. This can happen in different relationships, even within a marriage or long-term partnership. It can also happen in childhood. The harm can leave behind strong feelings of guilt, shame, and fear. Survivors might blame themselves for not stopping the event or for trusting the person who hurt them.

Sexual trauma can cause a sense of feeling unsafe in one's own body. It can lead to nightmares, flashbacks, and discomfort with any touch. Many survivors find it hard to share what happened, so they keep it inside. This can add to feelings of isolation and sadness. Finding a safe environment to talk or seeking professional help is often needed to reduce the effects of sexual trauma.

---

4. Combat Trauma

Combat trauma refers to the stress and harm that military personnel face in war or active duty situations. This might include seeing close friends wounded or killed, facing life-threatening attacks, and being in a constant state of high alert. People who have combat trauma might see themselves as strong and self-reliant, so they might not feel comfortable talking about fear or helplessness. Still, the memories of war can be very intense. Bomb explosions, gunfire, or loud sounds can trigger flashbacks.

Combat trauma can also lead to a sense of loss if a fellow service member does not survive. Feelings of guilt might arise if someone believes they should have saved a friend. Veterans might face difficulty readjusting to civilian life, especially if everyday noises or crowded places bring back memories of combat zones. This form of trauma can be quite complex and often needs targeted support and care.

---

5. Childhood Trauma

Childhood trauma can come from physical or emotional harm, neglect, or a lack of safety during early years. Children who face trauma may not understand what is happening. They might feel powerless or confused. If a caregiver is the one causing the harm, it can break the child's sense of trust. This can affect how they see themselves and how they form relationships later in life.

Childhood trauma can also happen if a child is in a household where there is drug abuse, violence, or chronic stress. The child might carry these experiences into adulthood. They can develop patterns of fear, anxiety, or emotional numbness. Early trauma can shape the way the brain grows, making it harder to handle stress in healthy ways. The child might struggle with school or behavior. Later in life, they might keep these coping problems if they do not receive help.

---

6. Complex Trauma

Complex trauma usually refers to repeated or long-lasting harm, especially during sensitive life stages. This might be ongoing physical or emotional abuse over months or years, often by someone the person relies on. Because of the repeated nature of the harm, the individual might feel like there is no safe way out. Over time, they might stop believing in their own worth or potential. Complex trauma can make people feel trapped, hopeless, and unsure of who they are.

Healing from complex trauma can be harder because the event is not a single incident. It is ongoing or repeated. The brain and body might adapt to always being in danger, making it harder to calm down or trust. Complex trauma might also lead to deep issues with self-image and relationships. Specialized therapy and strong support networks can be vital for those who have experienced complex trauma.

---

7. Secondary or Vicarious Trauma

You do not have to experience a harmful event yourself to face trauma. Sometimes, seeing or hearing about someone else's traumatic event can cause what is called secondary or vicarious trauma. Counselors, nurses, doctors, firefighters, and others who work with victims of tragedy can feel the weight of the stories they hear. Over time, this repeated contact with traumatic details can cause symptoms like sadness, worry, or intrusive thoughts.

Family members of people with PTSD can also face vicarious trauma. Constantly seeing their loved one upset might lead them to share that mental stress. They might develop their own nightmares or fears, even though they did not go through the event themselves. It is important to note that secondary trauma is real and should be taken seriously. Those who work in helping professions are urged to have resources to protect and care for their own well-being.

---

8. Medical Trauma

A person can also face trauma from medical procedures or serious health issues. A frightening diagnosis, a tough hospital stay, or treatments that cause pain can create lasting distress. People with chronic illnesses or who have gone through many hospital visits might feel overwhelmed. They might begin to have nightmares about hospitals or fear even small checkups. This can make it hard to get the care they need because they want to avoid triggers.

Medical trauma can sometimes be overlooked because it happens in a setting meant to help. But it can be shocking to feel powerless while undergoing painful treatments. The memory of the hospital can linger, and the person might panic the next time they see doctors, nurses, or machines that remind them of their experience.

---

9. Natural Disaster Trauma

Natural disasters like hurricanes, floods, earthquakes, and wildfires can leave people feeling unsafe. These events can destroy homes and take away the comforts of daily life. They can also separate families if someone gets hurt or must evacuate quickly. Even after it is over, the fear of another disaster can linger. The sound of strong wind or heavy rain might cause flashbacks.

People who go through such events might have trouble sleeping or feel anxious whenever weather conditions seem similar. They may also feel sad or shocked after losing their home or their community. It can be hard to move on from the idea that the environment they once trusted has become a threat.

---

10. Grief Trauma

Losing a loved one can be deeply upsetting. If the death was unexpected or violent, the sense of trauma can be even higher. The pain of loss can mix with regret or guilt, making a person feel emotionally raw. Grief is already tough to handle, and when the loss comes from a tragedy, it can feel unbearable.

A person might replay the final moments in their head, wishing they could have done something differently. They might feel overwhelmed by sadness, anger, or disbelief. While grief by itself is common, it can become traumatic if it involves shocking or horrifying details. In those cases, extra support can help the person cope with both the loss and the stress.

Why Different Types of Trauma Matter

Knowing the wide range of traumatic events is important because it helps people see that their feelings might be valid. Sometimes, a person might say, "Well, I have not been to war, so I can't have PTSD," or "I was never physically harmed, so what happened to me is not that bad." But everyone's response is personal. A single event can make a deep mark on one person, while another person might face multiple events and still not have the same reactions. Recognizing the various forms of trauma lets us be more understanding toward ourselves and others.

Trauma Does Not Always Fit Perfect Labels

These categories can give a general sense of what might cause trauma, but real life is not always so neat. A person can go through more than one type of trauma at the same time. They might face physical and emotional harm together, or experience a natural disaster while also grieving the loss of a loved one. Each person's life is unique, so it is not enough to say that one category alone explains everything.

Still, these types of trauma help us talk about and think about the problems that can come from extreme stress. They can guide professionals in figuring out which strategies might help and which forms of therapy might be most suitable. They also help family members, friends, and caregivers understand what the person is going through.

How Different Traumas Affect Coping

Each type of trauma can bring its own set of challenges. For instance, someone with a long history of emotional trauma might have trouble trusting others or feeling safe in relationships. Someone who faced a natural disaster might panic every time the weather changes. Understanding that these issues tie back to a person's traumatic event can reduce shame or self-blame. It can also guide the person to the right resources.

For example:

- A child who suffered repeated harm might need therapy that focuses on rebuilding a sense of safety and worth.
- A veteran with combat trauma might need treatment that deals with triggers related to loud noises and crowded settings.
- A car accident survivor might need special help to ride in or drive a car again.

All these different paths point to how personal trauma can be. Recognizing which category or categories apply can be the first step in finding the proper help.

Making Sense of Your Experience
It is possible that as you read through these types, you might notice that your past experiences fit more than one category. Maybe you had a near-fatal car accident (physical trauma) and also lost someone important in that accident (grief trauma). This can make things more complicated. One kind of trauma can add to another. That is why it is helpful to think about the different areas of your life that might be affected.

Thinking about the nature of your experience can also help you describe it better to counselors, doctors, or friends. Clarity allows others to see the full picture. It also lets you figure out what triggers might set off memories or fears. With this knowledge in hand, you can begin to plan steps toward feeling better.

Breaking the Silence
Many types of trauma can involve shame or embarrassment. People might feel afraid to speak up if their trauma came from a partner, family member, or someone in authority. Others might worry that no one will believe them. But staying silent often makes the pain grow bigger inside. Finding even one safe person—a friend, a counselor, a support hotline—can help reduce the weight. Talking about trauma may feel scary at first, but it is often a step toward relief.

For those who are not ready to speak with someone, writing or creating art can offer a way to express their pain. Some people find that writing down their thoughts helps them let go of some tension. Others might paint or draw images to show how they feel inside. Any healthy form of expression can be a way to release built-up emotions.

Why Understanding Trauma Matters

When we know more about different forms of trauma, we can be kinder to ourselves and others. We can see that a wide array of problems can be linked to events that happened long ago. Rather than just blaming someone for "being difficult," we can realize that they might be dealing with triggers that tie back to their trauma. This approach can lead to more compassion and patience.

It also reminds us that we do not have to face things alone. There are experts who specialize in certain areas of trauma. For instance, there are counselors who work with veterans, therapists who understand child abuse, or support groups for people who have faced a natural disaster. By learning about the different forms of trauma, we can find the specific help we need.

Moving Toward Getting Help

Different types of trauma can require different treatments, but they often share some of the same basic needs: a sense of safety, a chance to process feelings, and support from others. In the next chapters, we will look more at signs and symptoms, how trauma affects the body, and ways to handle triggers. By looking at all these aspects, we will gain a clearer view of how to move forward.

It is also important to remember that you do not have to wait until everything is really bad before asking for help. Even if you are not sure your experience counts as "bad enough," it can be useful to talk to someone you trust. You deserve to be heard and supported, no matter what type of trauma you have gone through.

Chapter 3: Signs and Symptoms

When someone has gone through a disturbing or harmful event, they might notice changes in how they feel, think, and act. These changes can sometimes suggest that they have Post-Traumatic Stress Disorder (PTSD) or another stress-related condition. While many people experience stress after something bad happens, PTSD is different because of the strength and length of its signs. In this chapter, we will talk in detail about the common signs and symptoms that can show up in people who have gone through trauma. We will also look at how these signs might show in adults, children, and older people, and how they can affect daily life. By recognizing these signs, people can figure out if they need help and learn where to get it.

---

1. Four Main Categories of Symptoms

Mental health professionals often group the signs of PTSD into four general groups:

1. **Intrusive symptoms**
2. **Avoidance symptoms**
3. **Negative changes in thoughts and mood**
4. **Changes in alertness and reactivity**

These groups can appear differently in each person. One individual might have many intrusive symptoms but fewer avoidance signs, while someone else might try hard to avoid everything related to the trauma. Recognizing these categories can help us see the big picture of PTSD and why it can be so hard to manage if a person does not get help.

1.1 Intrusive Symptoms

Intrusive symptoms are thoughts and memories of the bad event that come without warning or are hard to stop. They force themselves into a person's mind, sometimes in frightening or very vivid ways. They include:

- **Flashbacks**: A flashback makes someone feel as if they are living through the trauma again in real time. They might feel the same fear or pain they did during the event. Their heart may race, their hands might get sweaty, or they might struggle to breathe. These moments can be short or last for many minutes.

- **Bad dreams**: Sleep can be disrupted by dreams that replay the event or show similar fearsome situations. Sometimes these dreams are direct reflections of the trauma, but other times they are symbolic. A person might wake up frightened and have trouble going back to sleep.
- **Upsetting thoughts**: Even when a person is awake, they might have unwanted memories or mental pictures of what happened. A sight, sound, or smell that reminds them of the event can bring these thoughts to the surface.
- **Physical responses**: Along with these mental images, the body may respond with a racing heartbeat, tense muscles, or upset stomach. This reaction can happen quickly and feel overwhelming, as if danger is nearby.

Intrusive symptoms can make someone feel trapped. They might be working, spending time with loved ones, or trying to relax, and suddenly, the memory comes rushing back. This can be confusing and cause people to feel they have no control over their mind.

1.2 Avoidance Symptoms

Avoidance symptoms are actions or thoughts a person uses to stay away from anything linked to the traumatic event. This might involve clear decisions to avoid certain people or locations, or it might be more subtle, like shifting a conversation away from any reminder of the event. Examples include:

- **Staying away from reminders**: A person might not watch shows, read news, or go places that bring back painful memories. If someone's trauma was a car crash, they may refuse to drive or ride in cars.
- **Refusing to talk about it**: Many people with PTSD choose not to share details of what happened. They might change the topic whenever it comes up or become tense when asked about it.
- **Emotional numbing**: Some people avoid their own feelings by becoming numb. They push away any emotion that might be tied to the trauma. They may say they feel empty or disconnected.

While avoidance can give a short sense of safety, it can also limit a person's life. They might miss important events or lose friendships because they cannot face certain places or conversations. Over time, avoidance can shrink their world, adding sadness or loneliness to the original trauma.

1.3 Negative Changes in Thoughts and Mood

After going through a harmful event, many people find that their outlook on life changes. They might develop harsh or untrue beliefs about themselves or the world. These shifts can be strong and might look like:

- **Strong negative beliefs**: "I am a bad person," "The world is always dangerous," or "No one can be trusted." These beliefs might feel absolute and unshakable.
- **Blaming oneself or others**: Sometimes people believe they should have acted differently to stop the trauma. They might carry guilt, even if they had no real control.
- **Loss of interest**: Activities that used to bring joy may no longer seem fun. A person might withdraw from hobbies or friends, feeling that nothing matters.
- **Feeling cut off**: People with PTSD can feel detached from those around them. They might sense that nobody understands them. This can lead to loneliness and sadness.
- **Trouble feeling positive emotions**: Some might find it difficult to feel happy or hopeful. It can be as if part of their heart is locked away.

These changes in thinking and mood can affect a person's self-esteem and relationships. Close friends might notice that the person is sad or distant. Partners might feel shut out. Negative thoughts can also make it harder to seek help, as the person may believe that nothing can help them.

1.4 Changes in Alertness and Reactivity

Another core sign of PTSD is when the body stays in an ongoing state of alert, as if danger could appear at any moment. This can look like:

- **Being jumpy**: Even small noises or surprises can cause an extreme startle reaction.

- **Irritability or anger**: The person might snap at others or feel angry for no clear reason. This anger can show up suddenly and be hard to control.
- **Trouble sleeping**: Worries, nightmares, and overall tension can make it hard to fall asleep or stay asleep. Lack of rest can increase other issues like mood swings.
- **Reckless or risky behavior**: Some might drive too fast, misuse substances, or act on impulse. They may feel the need to do something intense to deal with their internal stress.
- **Difficulty concentrating**: Staying focused on tasks at school or work can be tough when the mind is on guard for threats.

These physical and behavioral changes come from a body that is used to being on high alert. It can exhaust a person and strain their relationships, as others might not understand why they are so edgy. Over time, constant alertness can also lead to health problems like headaches, muscle tension, or chronic fatigue.

2. Other Signs That Can Appear in PTSD

Beyond the main categories, there are other signs that can appear when someone is dealing with traumatic stress:

- **Emotional outbursts**: Sudden crying, shouting, or shaking due to overwhelming emotion.
- **Shame or guilt**: These emotions can be powerful if the person thinks they should have acted differently during the event or if they feel embarrassed about what they went through.
- **Low self-esteem**: They might see themselves as broken or weak because they cannot shake off their fears.
- **Physical problems**: Pain or tension in the body with no clear medical cause, stomach issues, or headaches may become frequent.
- **Changing view of life**: Someone might question past beliefs. For instance, they may lose faith in the idea that the world is good or that people are kind.

Not everyone will have all these signs, but noticing any of them might be a clue that something deeper is going on. Also, symptoms can vary in how strong they are from day to day or over time.

3. How Long Symptoms Last and When They Might Show Up

PTSD symptoms usually last more than a month and can persist for months or years if not addressed. Some people see signs right away, within a few days or weeks of the event. Others might not notice them until months or even years later. Triggers like anniversaries, smells, or discussions can set off memories that bring old pain to the surface.

Sometimes, people think they are fine right after the bad event. They keep going on with life. Then, something small reminds them of the trauma, and all the stress resurfaces. This delayed start can be confusing because they might not connect current symptoms with something that happened long ago. Recognizing that PTSD can wait before showing up helps people know that unexpected anxiety or distress might have a real cause tied to past events.

---

4. Signs of PTSD in Children

PTSD looks a little different in children. They might not talk about their feelings the same way adults do. Parents, teachers, or caregivers might have to watch for changes like:

- **New fears**: A child might develop specific worries that seem connected to the event. For example, if there was a home fire, the child might fear any flame.
- **Clinginess**: Young children might not want to be apart from parents or trusted adults. They might cry when they have to leave home.
- **Bedwetting or thumb-sucking**: If a child was already past these behaviors, going back to them can signal stress.
- **Acting out the trauma**: Kids sometimes replay the event during play. For instance, they might use toys to mimic a fight or a crash.
- **Trouble sleeping or nightmares**: Just like adults, children might face bad dreams or refuse to go to bed.
- **Anger or irritability**: A once easygoing child might have tantrums or mood swings.

Because children cannot always explain what is in their minds, adults might mistake these signs for just being "difficult." Understanding how trauma can look in children helps caregivers respond with patience and care.

5. Signs of PTSD in Teens

Teens are in a changing phase of life, so adding trauma to the mix can make things more complex. Some signs of PTSD in teens might mirror those in adults, such as flashbacks or avoidance. But teens might also:

- **Show more anger**: They might lash out at family or friends.
- **Struggle at school**: Grades might drop because they cannot focus, or they might skip class due to fear or shame.
- **Seek risky behavior**: Some teens might turn to substance misuse or unsafe actions to distract from their pain.
- **Withdraw from others**: They might stay in their room, ignore calls, or spend lots of time alone because they feel no one understands.
- **Display identity confusion**: Trauma can shake a teen's sense of who they are. They might experiment with different behaviors to cope.

Recognizing these changes can be crucial for helping teens find support early. If a parent or teacher sees a sharp change in behavior after a known bad event, it could be a signal to reach out to a counselor or mental health expert.

---

6. Signs of PTSD in Older Adults

Older adults can also face PTSD, especially if they have gone through wartime events, accidents, or the loss of loved ones. In some cases, they might have had symptoms for many years but never received help. As they retire or slow down in life, they may find they have more time to think about the past, which can bring back old memories. Some signs include:

- **Increased anxiety**: They might worry more about safety and health, refusing to leave home.
- **Physical complaints**: Headaches, stomach problems, or body pains can get worse when emotional stress is high.
- **Sadness or loneliness**: They might feel they cannot share their experiences with anyone, or they think it is too late to get help.
- **Withdrawal**: Some might isolate themselves from friends or family gatherings, feeling like no one can relate to them.

Caregivers and family members should be aware that older adults are not free from PTSD. Even if the event happened decades ago, the stress can remain if it was never addressed.

7. Effects on Daily Life

Living with strong symptoms of PTSD can affect nearly every part of a person's life:

1. **Work or school**: Concentration might be poor, or panic might keep the person from attending or performing well. They might struggle with tasks that were once easy.
2. **Relationships**: Friends and family might see a person pull away, or they might deal with sudden bursts of anger or sadness. Trust issues can cause fights or misunderstandings.
3. **Self-care**: A person might ignore healthy eating, exercise, or personal grooming. They might also overeat or oversleep to avoid their feelings.
4. **Leisure time**: Activities that once brought fun can seem pointless or stressful. A person might also avoid going out because it could lead to flashbacks.
5. **Physical health**: Chronic stress can lower the immune system, leading to more frequent illnesses. Headaches, body pain, or stomach issues might get worse when PTSD is untreated.

When these problems stack up, a person can feel trapped by the trauma. That is why noticing signs early is a key step toward finding relief.

---

8. How Symptoms Can Trick Someone

PTSD can cause a person to see danger everywhere. They might feel certain that disaster is just around the corner, or they might believe they are not worthy of help. Some of these "tricks" include:

- **Overgeneralizing**: After facing a single harmful event, a person might think every similar situation will end badly. For example, after a bad fall while hiking, they might decide that all outdoor activities are unsafe.
- **Catastrophic thinking**: A small hiccup in daily life can blow up into a huge fear. A minor sound at night might make them believe someone is breaking in.
- **Emotional reasoning**: If they feel terrified, they believe they must be in danger. Even if there is no real threat, the emotion feels like proof.
- **Self-blame**: They might accept full responsibility for the trauma, telling themselves they should have stopped it.

These ways of thinking can feed into each other, making PTSD stronger over time. Understanding these thought patterns can help a person see that the mind might be stuck in old fears.

---

9. Recognizing the Difference Between PTSD and Other Stress Reactions

Some people have mild or moderate stress after a tough situation, but it may not become PTSD. So how can someone tell the difference?

- **Length of time**: PTSD signs usually last a month or longer and do not fade much on their own.
- **Severity**: PTSD can deeply disrupt daily life. It can make it impossible to hold a job, keep up with schoolwork, or maintain relationships.
- **Type of symptoms**: While normal stress might include worry or sadness, PTSD involves powerful flashbacks, avoidance, and a constant sense of danger.

Only a qualified professional can diagnose PTSD. Still, if a person notices that their thoughts, feelings, or behaviors fit what we have outlined, it may be a sign that they need a mental health evaluation.

---

10. Why Early Identification Helps

The earlier a person notices PTSD symptoms, the sooner they can look for help. Waiting a long time can let those symptoms grow stronger. They can spread into more aspects of life, such as relationships or physical health. By identifying signs early, a person can:

1. **Reach out for professional guidance**: A therapist or counselor can offer tools to address flashbacks, avoidance, and negative thoughts.
2. **Build a support network**: Friends or loved ones can offer understanding and patience when they see what is going on.
3. **Adopt healthy habits**: Learning relaxation methods, practicing mindfulness, or exploring safe routines can lessen the grip of PTSD.
4. **Set realistic goals**: Early help can support a person in regaining control of daily tasks before the problem becomes too large.

11. When to See a Mental Health Professional

A good guideline is that if someone has trouble functioning at work, school, or home because of traumatic memories, they should seek help. If they cannot sleep, feel always on edge, or if they are pushing friends away for fear of being hurt, seeing a mental health professional could be key. There is no shame in wanting to feel better, and early care can prevent more suffering.

People might also consider help if they notice signs like panic attacks, thoughts of self-harm, or substance misuse as a way to handle nightmares or flashbacks. These signs can mean that the person is trying to cope in harmful ways. A professional can suggest better methods to manage these feelings.

---

12. The Role of Family and Friends in Spotting Symptoms

Sometimes, a person with PTSD might not see changes in themselves as clearly as others do. They might think they are just stressed or tired. Family members, friends, or coworkers might notice warning signs like:

- **Drastic changes in mood or behavior**
- **Frequent talk about feeling hopeless or guilty**
- **Refusal to go places or do activities they once enjoyed**
- **Flinching or reacting strongly to small triggers**
- **Trouble sleeping or looking tired all the time**

If someone close sees these signs, it might help to gently suggest professional help. It is important to be patient and avoid blaming the person. They might feel embarrassed or afraid of being judged. Simple reminders like "I'm here if you want to talk" or "I care about you and want you to feel better" can help.

---

13. Self-Awareness and Tracking Symptoms

One useful practice for those who suspect they have PTSD is to keep a daily journal of their thoughts and feelings. Each day, they can jot down any triggers, flashbacks, or nightmares they experienced. They can note what time it happened, where they were, and how they felt physically and emotionally. Over time, they might see patterns. For instance, they might discover that going to a certain part of town or hearing a specific type of music triggers their memories.

This information can be valuable when seeking professional help. A therapist might use these notes to plan treatment strategies, focus on coping skills for specific triggers, or suggest ways to handle unexpected reminders.

---

14. How Symptoms Can Change Over Time

PTSD symptoms do not always stay the same. They can shift depending on life circumstances, stress levels, or even changes in season:

- **Worsening during anniversaries**: When the date of the event comes around, a person might feel their flashbacks or anxiety increase.
- **Easing with support**: If someone finds a caring friend or therapist, they might see fewer nightmares or feel more at peace.
- **Returning after a new stress**: A new difficult event, even if unrelated, can stir up old pain. For example, losing a job could bring back memories of the trauma because of the stress.

Knowing that symptoms can go up and down helps a person prepare. They might realize that even if they are feeling better now, a trigger could bring some symptoms back. This is normal and does not mean they cannot keep going with healing efforts.

---

15. Special Considerations for Different Cultures

The signs of PTSD might look different depending on a person's cultural background or the beliefs of their family and community. In some cultures, people are more open about feelings, while in others, mental health issues are kept private. Some groups might describe symptoms in physical ways—like aches, weakness, or stomach problems—rather than saying "I am anxious" or "I am having flashbacks."

Being mindful of these differences can help someone find a therapist or support group that respects their background. It also helps family members understand that a loved one might not show the "typical" signs of PTSD. They could instead talk about how their body feels or mention fears that seem tied to cultural concerns.

16. The Danger of Ignoring Symptoms

If PTSD signs go unseen or ignored, they can become worse. A person might have:

- **Physical health issues**: Long-term stress can contribute to heart problems, high blood pressure, or frequent illness.
- **Higher risk of substance misuse**: Trying to quiet flashbacks or stress with drugs or alcohol can lead to addiction or other health problems.
- **Troubled relationships**: Friends or family might leave or become distant if they do not feel safe or supported.
- **Loss of personal goals**: Chronic symptoms can make it hard to keep a job or complete education plans.

All of these risks are serious. This is why learning to spot PTSD symptoms early and addressing them is so important.

17. Self-Test Questions

While only a professional can diagnose PTSD, here are some questions someone can ask themselves:

1. **Do I keep having intense or repeated memories of the event that I cannot control?**
2. **Am I going out of my way to avoid places, people, or activities that make me think of what happened?**
3. **Do I feel on guard or jumpy most of the time, even when things are calm?**
4. **Have I noticed changes in how I see myself or the world since the event?**
5. **Is my work, school, or home life suffering because of these issues?**

If the answer is "yes" to many of these, and it has lasted for more than a month, it is worth seeking a mental health evaluation. There is no need to wait until things get worse.

Chapter 4: How Trauma Affects the Body

When we discuss PTSD and trauma, we often focus on the emotional and mental parts. However, trauma also has a powerful impact on the body. When someone faces a harmful or scary event, their body reacts in a way meant to protect them from danger. After the event, these reactions can keep going, causing physical problems that add to the stress. In this chapter, we will talk about how the body's systems handle trauma and why these responses might continue. We will also look at the signs that appear in different parts of the body and strategies to address them.

1. The Body's Alarm System

Our bodies have built-in ways to help us survive threats. One of these is called the "fight, flight, or freeze" response. When we sense danger, our brain sends signals to release stress hormones like adrenaline and cortisol. These hormones make our heart beat faster, help us get more oxygen, and get the muscles ready to take action. This reaction is normal and can be life-saving in a real crisis.

However, in people with PTSD, this alarm system might stay on or get triggered by small reminders of the trauma. This can lead to chronic stress. Even when nothing is truly dangerous, the person's body responds as if danger is right there. That is why some people with PTSD sweat, shake, or feel their heart race when they hear a loud noise or see something that resembles the traumatic event.

2. The Role of Adrenaline and Cortisol

Adrenaline and cortisol are two main hormones that surge through the body in moments of stress:

1. **Adrenaline**: Causes immediate changes like faster heartbeat, sharper focus, and quick muscle responses. It readies a person to fight or run from danger.
2. **Cortisol**: Helps the body stay on alert by raising blood sugar for energy, reducing processes like digestion or growth that are not urgent for survival.

When someone is stuck in a PTSD cycle, the brain can trigger these hormones too often. Over time, high levels of cortisol can upset the body's balance. It can affect sleep, mood, and even the immune system. This can make a person feel constantly worn down or prone to illness.

---

3. Tension in Muscles

People dealing with trauma often have tense muscles. Their shoulders might be tight, their jaw might clench, or they could feel knots in their back. This tension can come from the body's attempt to guard itself against further harm. In a healthy situation, muscles tense briefly in response to danger, then relax when the danger passes. But in PTSD, the mind might keep telling the body that it is not safe, so the muscles stay locked.

Chronic muscle tension can lead to aches and pains, headaches, or problems like temporomandibular joint (TMJ) pain (jaw soreness). It also makes it harder to rest or sleep because the body never fully relaxes. Over time, this can lead to fatigue and reduce a person's ability to enjoy daily tasks.

---

4. Digestive Issues

The body cannot tell the difference between a real threat and a trigger when it comes to stress. During moments of danger, digestion is not a high priority. Blood flow is directed to the muscles and brain instead. If someone with PTSD remains in a stressed state, they might experience:

- **Loss of appetite**: Chronic fear or worry can make eating feel unimportant or even unpleasant.
- **Upset stomach**: Long-term stress can lead to cramping, diarrhea, or nausea.
- **Irritable bowel symptoms**: Some people develop ongoing problems with their bowels, which might flare up when their stress is high.
- **Acid reflux or heartburn**: Stress can make the stomach produce more acid, causing burning or discomfort.

These issues can be confusing. A person might see a doctor for stomach troubles and not realize that the root cause is ongoing stress from trauma.

5. Heart and Circulation Problems

When stress hormones flood the body, the heart beats faster to pump more blood. Blood pressure can rise as part of the fight-or-flight response. Over time, repeated episodes of high stress can strain the heart. Some possible effects include:

- **Increased blood pressure**: While short-term rises in blood pressure can be helpful in an emergency, constant stress can keep it high and raise the risk of heart problems.
- **Irregular heartbeat**: Some people feel palpitations or notice their heart skipping beats when they are anxious.
- **Long-term wear on arteries**: Continuous stress might contribute to plaque buildup or other heart-related concerns.

Keeping the body in this high-alert state for too long can put a person at greater risk for heart disease. That is why managing the physical side of stress is important for overall health.

6. Breathing Difficulties

Anxiety, panic, and flashbacks can also cause changes in breathing. A person might breathe faster or more shallowly during a PTSD-triggered moment. This can lead to:

- **Hyperventilation**: Taking rapid breaths can make someone dizzy or lightheaded.
- **Tightness in the chest**: The muscles around the chest might tense, making it feel harder to breathe.
- **Feelings of choking**: If the stress is severe, a person might feel like they cannot catch their breath at all.

These breathing problems can be scary and may feed into more fear. They can also make a person believe they are having a heart attack when it is actually an anxiety or panic response.

7. Sleep Disruption and Exhaustion

Trauma can interfere with a good night's sleep in several ways:

- **Nightmares**: A person may wake up suddenly, reliving the bad event. This can cause fear of going back to sleep.
- **Trouble falling asleep**: Being on high alert keeps the mind racing, making relaxation difficult.
- **Frequent waking**: Even small noises might rouse someone who is primed to detect any threat.

Lack of proper rest leads to daytime tiredness, difficulty thinking clearly, and mood swings. It can also weaken the immune system, making a person more prone to colds or other illnesses. Over time, severe insomnia can trigger more anxiety or depression, creating a vicious cycle.

---

8. Immune System Changes

Chronic stress from PTSD can affect the immune system. When the body is under threat, it tries to save energy for escaping danger, not for fighting germs or repairing tissues. As a result:

- **Frequent illnesses**: Some people get sick more often or take longer to recover from colds or infections.
- **Worsening of autoimmune conditions**: If someone already has an autoimmune issue, stress might make flare-ups more likely.
- **Slower healing**: Cuts, bruises, or other wounds might take more time to heal because the body is not devoting enough energy to repair.

This means that the aftermath of trauma can show up in frequent colds, allergies, or other health problems that seem unrelated to the original event.

---

9. Hormonal and Chemical Imbalances

In addition to cortisol, the body releases various hormones and chemicals in response to stress. If these remain high for long periods, they can upset the balance of neurotransmitters (chemical messengers in the brain). This imbalance can lead to:

- **Mood swings**: Rapid shifts between anger, sadness, or fear can happen when the brain's chemistry is uneven.
- **Trouble with memory and focus**: High stress can damage the brain's ability to store or recall new information.
- **Increased sensitivity to pain**: The body's ability to manage pain might decrease, making small aches feel worse.

By understanding these chemical changes, we see that trauma is not just mental. It is physical, too. That is why telling someone to "just stop thinking about it" does not help, since the entire body is involved.

10. The Mind-Body Connection in Trauma

Although we often talk about mind and body as if they are separate, they are closely linked. Emotions can affect physical processes, and physical problems can affect moods. When someone has PTSD, the mind might remember the trauma in clear or fuzzy ways, but the body can remember it in the form of muscle tension, faster heartbeat, or upset stomach. This mind-body link is key in understanding why trauma can be so powerful.

When a person feels afraid, the brain sends signals to the rest of the body to prepare for danger. If the event happened long ago but the mind still feels threatened, the body may stay in that prepared state. Over time, this can reshape how the brain and body communicate.

11. Long-Term Physical Health Risks

If untreated, the physical reactions to PTSD can lead to long-term health issues:

- **Chronic pain**: Neck, back, and joint pain can be made worse by tension and high levels of stress hormones.
- **Eating disorders**: Some people cope with stress by eating too much or too little.
- **Cardiovascular disease**: As noted, the heart and blood vessels suffer under chronic stress.
- **Mental health conditions**: Ongoing physical problems can lead to depression or deeper anxiety, especially if a person feels hopeless about getting better.

Recognizing these risks reminds us why it is vital to address both the emotional and physical sides of trauma.

---

12. Seeking Medical Assessment

People who suspect that PTSD is causing physical problems should consider talking to a medical professional. Doctors can check for things like high blood pressure or thyroid issues that might make anxiety or sleeplessness worse. They can also see if there are any nutritional gaps (like low vitamin levels) that might lead to tiredness or irritability.

Sometimes, addressing a physical problem can help lower stress. For instance, if a person's stomach pain is treated, they might worry less about it, and that can improve their overall mood. Working with both a doctor and a mental health specialist can lead to a more complete plan of care.

---

13. Techniques to Manage Physical Responses

A variety of methods can help calm the body after trauma:

1. **Breathing exercises**: Slow, deep breaths can tell the body it is safe. One simple method is to breathe in for four counts, hold for four, and breathe out for four.
2. **Progressive muscle relaxation**: This involves tensing then relaxing each muscle group in the body, starting from the toes up to the head. It teaches the body how to recognize and release tension.
3. **Physical movement**: Light stretching, walking, or gentle exercise can relieve built-up tension. Some people find activities like yoga (if available and comfortable) to be soothing, though any easy form of movement can help.
4. **Grounding techniques**: Focusing on the present moment by noticing five things you can see, four things you can touch, three things you can hear, and so on. This can reduce racing thoughts and bring awareness back to the body.
5. **Warm baths or showers**: Warm water can ease muscle tension and provide a sense of comfort.

These methods do not replace professional therapy, but they can support a person's efforts to manage physical stress. Over time, using these techniques can lower cortisol levels and help break the cycle of chronic alertness.

---

14. Importance of Rest and Nutrition

Taking care of the body through rest and good eating habits is vital for anyone dealing with PTSD. While it might sound simple, stress can make it hard to keep regular routines:

- **Setting a sleep schedule**: Going to bed and getting up at the same time each day helps regulate the body's clock.
- **Limiting caffeine or alcohol**: These can disturb sleep patterns or worsen anxiety if used too close to bedtime.
- **Choosing balanced meals**: Foods high in vitamins, minerals, and protein can help keep the body strong. Skipping meals or relying on junk food may add to the body's stress.
- **Staying hydrated**: Drinking enough water is key for overall well-being and can help manage headaches or fatigue.

When people with PTSD prioritize rest and nutrition, they give their body a stronger base to handle the extra stress. Sleep and good food will not erase trauma, but they can make the body more resilient.

---

15. Body-Based Therapies

Some therapies focus on the body's role in storing trauma. These approaches can help a person "release" the stress that might be trapped. Examples include:

- **Somatic experiencing**: A therapist helps the person notice and track physical sensations linked to trauma, then guides them to safely release tension.
- **Massage therapy**: Gentle touch can ease muscle tension and prompt relaxation, though it must be done in a way that feels safe to the person.
- **Movement or dance therapy**: Certain programs use guided motion to help people reconnect with their bodies and express stored feelings.

These therapies might be used along with talk therapy. While talk therapy addresses thoughts and emotions, body-based therapies deal with the physical side of trauma.

16. The Brain's Ability to Adjust

One piece of hopeful news is that the brain can change its pathways over time. This is sometimes called neuroplasticity. Even if a person's body has stayed in a stressed state for a while, learning coping methods and practicing them regularly can help rewire some of those fear pathways. By repeating calming techniques, positive self-talk, and safe experiences, a person can train the brain to lower the alarm response.

This does not mean recovery is automatic, but it shows that the body is not doomed to remain tense forever. With consistent steps, the stress response can become less intense.

17. Social Support and Physical Well-Being

Having supportive friends and family can also aid in physical well-being. Spending time with caring people can lower stress levels, release "feel-good" chemicals like oxytocin, and remind someone that they are not alone. Social activities can include calm get-togethers, shared meals, or simple walks in the park.

Feeling safe with others can help the body relax. Laughter, conversation, or just sitting quietly with someone you trust can tell the nervous system that there is no immediate danger. Over time, this sense of safety can reduce symptoms and promote better health.

18. Warning Signs That Need Quick Medical Help

Sometimes the stress on the body can lead to severe problems. It is important to seek medical care quickly if someone with PTSD notices:

- **Chest pain or tightness**: This could be a sign of heart trouble.
- **Severe dizziness or fainting**: Could show problems with blood pressure or oxygen supply.
- **Uncontrolled bleeding or injuries**: If stress leads to unsafe behaviors or self-harm, immediate help is needed.
- **High fever or serious infection**: A weakened immune system might make infections worse.

While not every ache or pain is an emergency, it is wise to pay attention to new or worsening symptoms. Letting a doctor know about one's PTSD can help them provide better, more informed care.

---

19. Rebuilding a Sense of Safety in the Body

Trauma can make a person feel that their own body is not a safe place to be. They might distrust what they feel, or they might try to disconnect from bodily sensations. Rebuilding trust in the body can be a slow but important process. Some helpful ideas include:

- **Gentle self-massage**: Rubbing your hands or shoulders calmly can help you reconnect with your body in a safe way.
- **Mindful movement**: Simple stretches where you pay attention to how your muscles feel can restore a sense of control.
- **Creative expression**: Activities like painting, making crafts, or playing an instrument can shift focus from fear to creation, reminding you that the body can do more than just hold tension.

By taking small steps to feel safer in their body, a person can move toward a healthier relationship with their physical self.

Chapter 5: Finding Professional Help

When dealing with Post-Traumatic Stress Disorder (PTSD) or deep trauma, finding a professional who can offer the right kind of help can make a big difference. Many people feel nervous or confused when they think about seeing a counselor, therapist, or doctor. They might not know where to look or which kind of treatment is best. This chapter will explain the different types of mental health professionals, how to select one, and what to expect when you begin this important process. We will also talk about common treatments, possible medications, and ways to handle the cost or practical barriers. By gaining clear information, you can move toward getting care that can make life feel more steady and manageable.

---

1. Recognizing the Need for Professional Support

You might decide you need professional help if you notice that your symptoms of trauma or PTSD are getting in the way of daily life. Here are some common signs:

1. **Ongoing flashbacks or nightmares**: These unwanted images continue to disturb your sleep or thoughts, no matter what you try on your own.
2. **Strong emotional reactions**: You might have intense anger, sadness, or fear that lasts longer than a few weeks or months.
3. **Problems at work or school**: It becomes hard to focus or finish tasks. You might miss days or struggle to keep up with your usual responsibilities.
4. **Trouble connecting with others**: Relationships might suffer because you feel on edge or avoid people you love.
5. **Risky coping methods**: You might find yourself misusing alcohol or other substances to quiet the pain.

Needing help is not shameful. It is a wise decision when you realize that your mental and physical health are at risk. Professionals who focus on trauma can offer a safe space to talk and can teach proven skills to handle the stress.

---

2. Types of Mental Health Professionals

Not all mental health providers have the same training or offer the same treatments. Here are some common professionals you might come across:

1. **Psychiatrists**: These are medical doctors who focus on mental health. They can diagnose conditions, provide therapy, and prescribe medications if needed. They spend time in medical school and then do specialty training in psychiatry.
2. **Psychologists**: They usually hold a doctoral degree (Ph.D. or Psy.D.) in psychology. They can diagnose and provide various therapy methods. They typically do not prescribe medications (in most places), but they can work closely with other medical professionals if medication might help.
3. **Licensed Counselors or Therapists**: Professionals such as Licensed Professional Counselors (LPC), Licensed Clinical Social Workers (LCSW), and Marriage and Family Therapists (LMFT) have graduate-level training in counseling or social work. They can diagnose and treat many mental health problems, using talk-based methods.
4. **Clinical Social Workers**: They hold a master's or doctoral degree in social work and focus on helping individuals navigate personal or societal problems. They can provide therapy, case management, and help connect people to community resources.
5. **Nurse Practitioners in Mental Health**: Some nurse practitioners have advanced training in mental health care. They can prescribe medication in many areas, provide counseling, and monitor a person's overall health.

Each type of professional has a unique way of helping. What matters most is finding someone qualified to work with people who have trauma or PTSD. Look for words like "trauma-informed" or "experience in PTSD treatment" in their descriptions.

---

3. Common Approaches to Therapy

Different methods can help people deal with trauma. Below are some that have been studied for PTSD and related conditions:

1. **Cognitive Behavioral Therapy (CBT)**: This style focuses on how your thoughts affect your emotions and actions. A therapist might help you notice unhelpful thoughts and replace them with more balanced ones.
2. **Eye Movement Desensitization and Reprocessing (EMDR)**: EMDR uses guided eye movements or other forms of bilateral (two-sided) stimulation while the person recalls parts of the traumatic event. Over time, this can reduce how frightening the memory feels.

3. **Prolonged Exposure Therapy**: This involves safely revisiting the trauma memory or related triggers in a controlled way. By doing this gradually, the person may learn that these cues are not harmful in the present.
4. **Trauma-Focused Therapy for Children**: This can include play therapy or other activities that help children express feelings. Therapists who work with kids often adapt standard treatments to be more child-friendly.
5. **Group Therapy**: Some people find it helpful to share their experiences with others who have faced similar events. A trained professional usually leads these sessions to keep them safe and respectful.

It is important to note that these approaches are not "one size fits all." Different methods help different people. A conversation with a professional can guide you in picking a method that feels right.

---

4. Medication Options

Sometimes, doctors or nurse practitioners suggest medication to manage PTSD or anxiety. Medications do not erase memories, but they can ease symptoms such as:

- **Anxiety and panic**
- **Sad or depressed mood**
- **Trouble sleeping**
- **Irritability and anger**

Typical medications might include:

1. **Antidepressants (SSRIs, SNRIs)**: These can help balance chemicals in the brain that affect mood and anxiety.
2. **Anti-anxiety medications**: While these can reduce intense fear or panic, they may carry risks if used long-term (some can be habit-forming).
3. **Beta-blockers**: Sometimes used to reduce the physical signs of stress, like a racing heart.
4. **Sleep aids**: If nightmares or insomnia are severe, certain prescriptions might be used for a short time.

Deciding to take medication is personal. Some people do very well with therapy alone, and others find that medication plus therapy is best. If you are unsure, talk to a psychiatrist or other prescriber about the pros and cons. It is also wise to mention any other medicines or supplements you use so that the professional can avoid harmful interactions.

5. Finding the Right Person for You

Picking a mental health professional can feel overwhelming. Here are a few tips:

1. **Ask for recommendations**: You can start by talking to your general doctor, who might know local therapists or psychiatrists skilled in trauma care. You can also ask trusted friends or family members if they have had good experiences with anyone.
2. **Check professional directories**: Many areas have mental health organization websites where you can filter providers by specialty, location, and insurance acceptance.
3. **Read their background**: Look at the professional's website or bio. Do they mention working with trauma survivors? Do they list approaches like EMDR, CBT, or other proven treatments?
4. **Ask questions**: When you first talk to a provider by phone or in person, feel free to ask about their experience with PTSD. You might also want to know their approach to treatment, fees, scheduling, or communication style.
5. **Trust your instincts**: You do not have to stay with the first person you see if it does not feel right. It is okay to look for someone else if you feel uncomfortable or if their style does not match what you need.

6. Dealing with Cost and Insurance

Cost is often a barrier. Therapy sessions and psychiatric visits can be expensive, and not all insurance plans cover them fully. However, there are options:

- **Insurance networks**: If you have insurance, see which mental health providers are "in-network." This often means lower out-of-pocket costs.
- **Sliding scales**: Some clinics or individual providers offer fees based on what you can afford.
- **Community health centers**: These centers sometimes provide counseling for free or at reduced rates.

- **Employer programs**: Some workplaces have assistance plans that include mental health benefits.
- **Student services**: If you attend school or college, there might be on-campus counseling at no extra cost.

Try to ask providers directly about payment choices. Many professionals understand that therapy can be hard to afford, and they may offer suggestions to help you get care.

---

7. Confidentiality and Privacy

Therapy sessions are typically private. Professionals must follow rules to keep your information confidential. However, there are a few exceptions:

- If you say you might harm yourself or someone else, a therapist may need to seek help.
- If there is suspicion of child or elder harm, they may have to report it to the authorities.

Besides these exceptions, what you share in therapy stays there. This can help you feel safer being open and honest about what you have gone through.

---

8. What to Expect at Your First Appointment

You might feel nervous before your first session. That is normal. During the first visit, the professional will likely:

1. **Ask about your reasons for seeking help**: They will want to know what is happening in your life and what problems you want to address.
2. **Gather your history**: This might include any past trauma, medical issues, and other mental health concerns. They may also ask about your upbringing or family background if relevant.
3. **Explain how they work**: They will describe their approach to therapy, how often you will meet, and what you can hope to gain from it.
4. **Encourage questions**: You can ask about their experience with clients who have had similar challenges. It is also fine to discuss fees, how to reach them between sessions, and how long treatment might last.

If you decide the fit is good, you will plan future appointments. If not, you can kindly let them know you want to look elsewhere. A good provider will respect your choice.

---

9. Stigma and Fear About Seeking Help

Some people worry about what friends or family will say if they begin therapy. Others might fear being judged or labeled as "crazy." However, seeking help for emotional health is no different from seeing a doctor for physical pain. Trauma is not your fault, and therapy is simply a tool to manage its effects.

If someone around you does not understand, it can help to explain that therapy teaches healthy ways to handle stress. If you do not feel comfortable sharing, that is your right. Your therapy sessions are personal, and you have no duty to tell anyone unless you want to.

---

10. Handling Setbacks or Slow Progress

It is rare for symptoms to vanish right away after the first few sessions. Healing can take time, and it might involve ups and downs. You might feel better for a while and then find yourself struggling again, especially if something in life triggers old memories. This does not mean that therapy is not working. It often signals that you are digging deeper into what caused your distress. Here are some tips to handle setbacks:

- **Share openly with your provider**: Tell them if you are feeling worse or if certain methods are not helping. They can adjust the approach.
- **Set realistic goals**: Ask yourself what you hope to improve in the short term. Maybe it is sleeping through the night or handling a specific trigger. Long-term goals can come later.
- **Reward small steps**: If you go to therapy regularly or practice new skills, recognize that as progress.
- **Seek additional support**: Sometimes, a support group or extra sessions might help if you are going through a rough patch.

---

11. Exploring Other Helpers

Therapists and psychiatrists are not the only ones who can assist you:

1. **Pastoral or spiritual counselors**: If faith or spirituality is important to you, you might find help in talking to a leader you trust. Some are trained to provide counseling.
2. **Peer support specialists**: These are individuals who have faced mental health problems themselves and learned ways to cope. They are trained to support others going through similar experiences.
3. **Occupational therapists**: Sometimes, trauma affects a person's ability to complete daily tasks. Occupational therapists can help you develop routines that reduce stress.
4. **Local support agencies**: Organizations in your community might offer crisis hotlines, safe houses, or groups for survivors of specific traumas.

Using multiple forms of help can provide a well-rounded plan. For instance, you might see a therapist weekly, talk to a peer specialist in between, and attend a group session once a month.

---

12. Questions to Ask a Potential Provider

Before you commit to therapy, you might want to make sure you and the provider are a good fit. You could ask:

- **Do you have experience working with people who have been through similar events?**
- **What is your treatment method for trauma or PTSD?**
- **How long are your typical sessions, and how often would we meet?**
- **What is your policy if I need to cancel or reschedule?**
- **What kind of payment do you accept, and do you offer a sliding scale?**

Asking these questions helps you avoid surprises and gives you a feel for the provider's style and attitude.

---

13. Online and Telehealth Options

In many regions, telehealth services have grown, allowing people to have video or phone sessions with mental health professionals. This can be helpful if:

- **You live far from a city**: Online options save the time and cost of traveling.
- **You have mobility challenges**: If leaving home is difficult, video calls can be more practical.
- **You feel unsafe going out**: Triggers or fears might keep you from wanting to visit an office in person.

Telehealth can still be effective for talk-based methods like CBT or counseling. Make sure the therapist is licensed in your state or region (if required) and that they provide secure, private video sessions.

---

14. Preparing for Therapy to Succeed

Your attitude going into therapy can shape how helpful it is. Some preparation tips:

1. **Stay open-minded**: It might feel strange at first to share personal events with someone you do not know. Try to remain open to the process.
2. **Be honest**: If you hold back important details, therapy might be less effective. Your counselor needs accurate information to help.
3. **Practice at home**: If you learn a method for dealing with stress, set aside time to do it outside of sessions.
4. **Keep track**: Some people find it useful to keep notes or a journal. Write down the things you talk about in therapy and the suggestions you receive. This makes it easier to remember and use the strategies.

---

15. Support Groups and Group Programs

Support groups are not a replacement for one-on-one therapy, but they can be a strong addition. Many groups meet weekly or monthly, either in person or online. They can help you:

- **Feel less alone**: Hearing others talk about their challenges can remind you that people share similar experiences.
- **Pick up new ideas**: Members may offer practical hints that worked for them.
- **Practice sharing**: If it is hard for you to talk about trauma, a group setting can be a first step in a caring environment.

If you decide to try a group, make sure it has a leader who can keep discussions respectful and supportive. Groups can focus on specific types of trauma (like natural disasters or childhood issues) or be open to anyone with PTSD.

16. Handling a Crisis

In a crisis—say you feel unsafe with your thoughts or you are worried you might harm yourself—do not wait for your next therapy appointment. Call emergency services or a trusted crisis hotline right away. Examples of times you might need quick help include:

- Feeling like you cannot stop harmful actions toward yourself
- Believing you might harm someone else because you feel out of control
- Seeing or hearing things that scare you to the point of panic

Many countries have emergency numbers, and some areas have mental health hotlines. Some hospitals also have urgent psychiatric care. Your safety is always the first concern.

17. Keeping an Eye on Your Progress

As you continue in therapy or medication, it helps to observe improvements or changes in symptoms. This might include:

- **Fewer nightmares** or less disturbing content when you sleep
- **Less fear** when exposed to mild triggers
- **Better mood** or an ability to cope with stress without losing control
- **Stronger relationships** with friends or family because you feel more open
- **Improved self-esteem** as you realize trauma does not define you

If you do not notice any positive changes after several weeks or months, consider talking to your provider about adjusting the approach. They may suggest different techniques or refer you to another professional who specializes in a method that might suit you better.

18. Combining Professional Help with Self-Care

Professional help is crucial for many people, but it often works best when paired with daily actions that support mental health. Some ways to supplement therapy include:

1. **Building regular routines**: Regular sleep, eating, and exercise can help stabilize your body's stress response.
2. **Practicing calming methods**: If your therapist teaches breathing exercises or visualization, use them at home.
3. **Staying in touch**: Reach out to supportive friends or family, so you do not feel isolated.
4. **Doing low-stress activities**: Activities like simple crafts, nature walks, or listening to soothing music can help you unwind.

These steps can keep you from relying on therapy sessions alone. You become an active partner in your own progress.

---

19. Overcoming Barriers to Getting Help

Many issues can stand in the way of finding professional help:

- **Fear or shame**: Feeling judged or embarrassed can keep people away. But mental health is like physical health—professionals are there to help, not to judge.
- **Transportation or distance**: Some people live in remote areas. Telehealth services might solve this challenge.
- **Cultural misunderstandings**: In some cultures, mental health concerns are not widely discussed. Looking for a provider familiar with your background can help.
- **Language issues**: If English (or the main language in your area) is not your first language, try to find a provider who speaks your language or who can provide interpretation.

Working around these barriers may take extra steps, but it is possible. The positive change you can gain often outweighs the trouble of getting past these obstacles.

Chapter 6: Stress Management Methods

Life can bring many stressors, but these can feel heavier if you are living with PTSD or the after-effects of a traumatic event. Beyond therapy and medical help, stress management skills can help you stay calm and reduce triggers. Using these methods does not remove the past, but they can give you greater control over your response when stress arises. This chapter covers practical ways to manage daily tension and emotional overload. These methods are meant to support, rather than replace, professional help.

1. Understanding Why Stress Management Is Important

Stress is your body's alarm system letting you know something might need attention. After trauma, that alarm might go off too often or at the wrong times. The goal of stress management is not to erase stress entirely, because some stress is normal and even helpful. Instead, the aim is to handle it in healthy ways. Benefits of managing stress include:

- **Better focus**: When your mind is less overwhelmed, you can pay attention to work, family, and personal interests.
- **Improved mood**: Lowering stress might help reduce anger, anxiety, or sadness.
- **Physical wellness**: Chronic stress can harm the body. Managing it can lessen muscle tension, headaches, or stomach problems.
- **More confidence**: Knowing you can calm yourself if a trigger appears can help you feel less powerless.

2. Identifying Your Triggers and Stressors

Before you can manage stress, it helps to know what causes it. Triggers can be anything that brings back memories or feelings tied to the trauma. Stressors can also include everyday issues like bills, deadlines, or family arguments. Some ways to identify them include:

1. **Keep a log**: Write down any events, places, or conversations that made you feel stressed or caused a surge of upsetting emotions.

2. **Notice body signs**: Stress often shows up physically—sweaty palms, tense muscles, or a tight chest. When you feel these signs, think about what might have caused them.
3. **Observe emotional shifts**: If your mood drops suddenly or you feel panic, recall what happened right before. Was there a noise, a smell, a certain date, or a particular worry on your mind?

Naming your triggers is the first step. Once you know them, you can make a plan to handle them or, in some cases, avoid them.

---

3. Time Management and Goal Setting

Everyday stress can add to your PTSD symptoms, so learning to organize tasks can bring a sense of control:

- **Make lists**: Write down what needs to get done and put the most important tasks at the top.
- **Break tasks into steps**: Large projects can feel overwhelming. Cutting them into smaller tasks can reduce the feeling of pressure.
- **Set clear deadlines**: If possible, give each task a timeframe. Even if it is flexible, it helps to have a target.
- **Use reminders**: Put notes on a calendar or set phone alerts. This helps your mind relax because you know you have a system in place.

When you manage your time, you reduce the chaos that can intensify your sense of being overwhelmed. Even small steps can lower stress levels.

---

4. Physical Activities

Moving your body can release tension and has been shown to help balance stress hormones. You do not need to do intense exercise to feel benefits. Here are some simple options:

1. **Gentle walking**: A short walk around your neighborhood or a nearby park can clear your head.
2. **Light stretching**: Spending a few minutes stretching your arms, legs, and back can relieve muscle tension.

3. **Easy aerobic routines**: If you have access to free online videos or community classes, you can try low-impact exercises.
4. **Dancing**: If it feels comfortable, you can put on music at home and move in a way that feels good.

Physical activities help the body process stress. They can also distract from swirling thoughts, at least for a little while.

---

5. Breathing and Relaxation Exercises

A calm breathing method can send signals to your nervous system that it is time to relax. Below are a few ways to do this:

- **Square breathing**: Inhale for a count of four, hold your breath for four, exhale for four, and pause again for four. Picture a square as you do each step.
- **Belly breathing**: Place a hand on your stomach. Inhale slowly through your nose, feeling your stomach rise. Exhale gently, noticing the stomach fall.
- **Calming images**: While you breathe slowly, imagine a peaceful place or a soothing color. Let the sense of calm fill your body.

If done regularly, these exercises can become a reliable tool to manage panic or sudden anxiety.

---

6. Mindful Awareness

Being mindful means paying close attention to the present moment without judging your thoughts or emotions. It can pull you away from dwelling on scary memories or worries about the future. Here are simple mindful activities:

1. **Mindful eating**: Take a small bite of food. Notice its texture, smell, and taste. Pay attention to how it feels in your mouth before swallowing.
2. **Sensory focus**: Look around the room and silently list five things you see, four things you can touch, three things you can hear, two you can smell, and one you can taste (or imagine tasting).

3. **Body scan**: Close your eyes and slowly move your focus from your toes to your head, noticing sensations or tension along the way.

Mindfulness does not require special equipment. It just needs a bit of time and willingness to pay close attention to the here and now.

7. Balancing Activity and Rest

Some people with trauma may avoid being alone with their thoughts, so they keep busy all day. Others might feel so drained that they do not want to leave the house. Both extremes can add stress. Finding a middle ground is key:

- **Plan breaks**: Schedule short breaks during the day to rest your mind, even if it is just for five minutes.
- **Create a comfortable space**: If you need alone time, set up a calm corner with pillows, soft lighting, or calming music.
- **Avoid overbooking**: Learn to say "no" when you are at your limit. Taking on too many obligations can spike stress levels.

Striking a balance gives your body time to recover from tension, while also keeping you connected to everyday life activities.

8. Creative Outlets

Expression through art, writing, or other creative forms can help process tough emotions. You do not need to be an artist or writer to benefit:

1. **Drawing or painting**: Let colors or shapes show how you feel. You can paint something abstract if direct images are too painful.
2. **Journaling**: Some people write down their thoughts or describe triggers and their reactions. Others might list what they are thankful for or write supportive words to themselves.
3. **Music**: Listening to calm tunes or creating your own (even simple humming) can shift your focus away from negative thoughts.
4. **Craft projects**: Making something with your hands—like knitting, pottery, or collage—can calm a racing mind.

Creative efforts can offer a sense of accomplishment and a channel for feelings that may be hard to express with words alone.

9. Self-Compassion and Healthy Self-Talk

Harsh self-criticism can make stress worse. Instead, try these ideas:

- **Use kind words**: When you notice self-blame, replace it with gentle phrases like, "I'm doing the best I can right now."
- **Accept limits**: You may not be able to handle as much stress as before the trauma. That is okay. Respect your current limits while still moving toward small improvements.
- **Acknowledge growth**: If you manage to do something that used to be too scary, even if it is a small step, remind yourself that this shows progress.

Being fair and understanding with yourself can reduce inner pressure. It is a way to calm the mind instead of fueling self-doubt.

10. Planning for Unexpected Stress

Life can throw surprises at any time, which can trigger anxiety or flashbacks. It helps to have a basic plan:

1. **Have a grounding method ready**: If something unexpected happens, you might immediately do a breathing exercise or a mental check-in.
2. **Create a calming kit**: Fill a small box or bag with items that help you calm down, such as a stress ball, a comforting photo, or scented lotion.
3. **Set up a text or call group**: Ask a couple of trusted friends or family members if you can contact them in tense moments.
4. **Know your safe places**: Identify a few spots (like your car, a nearby restroom, or a quiet corner) where you can step away if you start to feel overwhelmed in public.

Having a plan in place can lower the fear of being caught off-guard by triggers.

11. Healthy Boundaries with Others

Interacting with people can be complicated when you have PTSD. Setting boundaries can protect your mental health:

- **Say "no" when needed**: If a gathering or event is likely to be too stressful, it is okay to decline.
- **Limit negative input**: If certain friends or relatives only bring drama or arguments, keep contact limited or focus on safer subjects.
- **Explain your needs**: You do not have to share every detail of your trauma, but you can say, "I'm working on handling stress, so I need some space right now."

Boundaries help you feel more secure in relationships. You remain in control of how much you interact and on what terms.

---

12. Pets and the Comfort They Provide

Animals can offer support without judgment. Many people find it soothing to spend time with a pet:

- **Companionship**: Pets can make you feel less alone. They are often sensitive to your emotions and can provide warmth or calm.
- **Routine**: Feeding, walking, or grooming a pet can structure your day and give a sense of purpose.
- **Stress relief**: Studies show that petting an animal can lower blood pressure and release relaxing chemicals in the body.

Even if you cannot own a pet, spending time with a friend's animal or volunteering at a shelter may bring comfort.

---

13. Limiting Overexposure to Media

The news or social media can be filled with upsetting stories, which can raise stress for someone with PTSD. While staying informed is good, consider:

- **Setting time limits**: Decide how long you will watch or read the news, and stick to it.

- **Choosing sources carefully**: Look for news outlets or online groups that focus on positive or balanced content rather than shocking images.
- **Silencing notifications**: Constant alerts can increase tension. Turn them off for periods of time.

Managing your media intake can reduce unneeded anxiety that might pile on top of existing stress.

---

14. Simple Grounding Methods for Daily Use

We touched on mindfulness earlier, but here are a few more grounding tips to use when you feel stress creeping up:

1. **5-4-3-2-1 method**: Name five things you see, four you can touch, three you can hear, two you can smell, and one you can taste.
2. **Touch an object and focus on it**: It might be a rock, a piece of fabric, or anything close by. Notice its texture, weight, and temperature.
3. **Count backward**: Start from a certain number (like 30) and count backward by threes or twos.

These quick actions help your mind slow down and reconnect with the present moment instead of getting lost in anxious thoughts.

---

15. Keeping a Calm Environment

If possible, shape your home or workspace into a calmer place:

- **Soft lighting**: Bright or flickering lights might trigger anxiety.
- **Reduced clutter**: Messy areas can make stress worse because they remind you of undone tasks.
- **Comforting scents**: If you like certain smells, use them in candles or diffusers (but be mindful if strong scents trigger you).
- **Background music**: Soft, rhythmic music can soothe the mind, although it is best to avoid anything that reminds you of bad events.

Small changes in your environment can ease the constant stress that comes from feeling on edge.

16. Seeking Social Support

While boundaries are important, so is having a circle of people who understand or care. Some ways to find support:

- **Friends and family**: You might lean on a close friend who listens without judgment.
- **Support groups**: Local or online groups for trauma survivors can allow sharing in a safe space.
- **Online forums**: If in-person groups are too intimidating, reading posts from others with PTSD can reassure you that you are not alone (but be careful to avoid unhealthy or disrespectful spaces).
- **Recreational clubs**: Joining a low-pressure hobby group or community class can help you build social ties without the focus on trauma.

Connecting with others, even in small steps, can help reduce feelings of isolation and boost hope.

---

17. Positive Distractions

Sometimes, you need to shift your focus quickly away from swirling thoughts:

- **Puzzles or word games**: They demand enough attention to keep your mind occupied.
- **Video games**: Simple puzzle or adventure games can provide a short break from anxious thinking.
- **Watching gentle shows**: Pick content that is funny or uplifting rather than violent or sad.
- **Cooking or baking**: Following a recipe step by step can calm the mind.

Positive distractions are not a permanent fix, but they can help you catch your breath before going back to any deeper issues.

---

18. Tracking Your Stress Levels

Similar to keeping a log of triggers, you can track your daily stress level using a simple scale from 1 to 10. Write down:

- **What was happening** when you felt your stress rise
- **Your thoughts and feelings** at that time
- **The action you took** (such as breathing exercises)
- **How it turned out** (did stress go down, stay the same, or increase?)

Over time, patterns might appear. You might see that certain methods work better for you, or certain times of day are tougher. This information can guide you to make changes.

---

19. Avoiding Unhelpful Shortcuts

Some stress relief methods might work temporarily but cause more harm later, such as:

- **Using alcohol or drugs**: While they may numb feelings at first, they often increase anxiety or create addiction problems.
- **Overspending or gambling**: These actions can distract from pain but lead to financial trouble and guilt.
- **Unhealthy relationships**: Clinging to someone just because they distract you from your thoughts can end poorly if the relationship is not supportive.

It is better to practice safe and sustainable stress management, even if it takes longer to feel the effects.

Chapter 7: Building Helpful Connections

When someone is dealing with Post-Traumatic Stress Disorder (PTSD) or strong trauma, having caring and understanding people around can make life feel safer. Building connections does not have to be complicated or time-consuming. Sometimes, a single trusted friend or family member can ease the weight of stress. In this chapter, we will look at why support from others matters, ways to form and keep connections, and steps to create a network that truly helps. We will also cover how to handle situations where the people around you might not understand trauma, as well as how to protect yourself from unhelpful or harmful relationships. The goal is to see how strong, kind bonds can lighten the pain of PTSD and foster a sense of belonging.

---

1. Why Connections Matter

Humans usually do better when they have at least a few supportive people around. This can include relatives, friends, coworkers, or neighbors. For someone facing PTSD, connections can:

1. **Ease feelings of loneliness**: Traumatic events can leave a person feeling alone or misunderstood. Having someone to talk to eases the sense of isolation.
2. **Offer practical help**: Supportive friends might help drive you to therapy, handle household tasks on days when you feel overwhelmed, or watch your children during tough moments.
3. **Lower stress levels**: A calm chat over the phone or a friendly text message can reduce tension in the mind and body.
4. **Remind you of hope**: Loved ones can see positive things about you that you might miss. They can encourage you when you feel down or anxious.

When we speak of connections, we do not mean that you need a huge group of friends or an ongoing social event. Even one or two caring individuals can make a big difference.

---

2. Deciding Whom to Trust

Many people with PTSD have trouble trusting others. This might stem from being hurt by someone or feeling that no one can understand their pain. Still, forming trust with the right individuals can offer healing. Some guidelines to consider:

1. **Check their actions**: A person who respects your limits, keeps your secrets, and is kind to you even when times are rough is likely trustworthy.
2. **Notice how you feel**: If you feel safe or calm after talking with someone, that is a good sign. If you always feel tense or ashamed, that person might not be right for close sharing.
3. **Start small**: You do not have to share your entire story at once. See how the other person responds to small pieces of information. If they react kindly, you might open up more slowly.
4. **Stay aware of pushy behavior**: If someone pressures you to talk when you are not ready, that might be a red flag. True support comes with patience.

Some individuals find it easier to trust a professional counselor first. Others share with a close friend or a relative. The key is to choose people who help you feel safer, not more vulnerable.

---

3. Friends and Family: Helping Them Understand

Some friends or family members might not know much about trauma or PTSD. They might say unhelpful things like "Just get over it" or "It was in the past—why are you still upset?" These remarks can hurt. However, sometimes people simply do not know better. You can try:

1. **Giving clear examples**: You might say, "When I hear loud bangs, my heart races, and I feel like I'm back in that situation. It's not just a random worry."
2. **Sharing reliable resources**: Offer articles or books that explain PTSD in simple terms. This helps loved ones see it is not about being weak.
3. **Explaining triggers**: If certain things or places make you panic, let your friend or family member know. Ask them to avoid bringing up those topics or to help you feel safe if a trigger appears.
4. **Suggesting ways to help**: A loved one may not know how to be supportive. You might say, "It helps if you can sit with me when I'm upset and not try to solve everything right away. Just listen."

Not everyone will react kindly, but many people do want to help if they understand how. It can take time for them to adjust. Keep in mind you do not have to tell everyone your full story; you can share what you feel comfortable sharing.

4. Building Support Outside of Family

Sometimes family members cannot be the primary support because they might be part of the trauma or they may not be emotionally available. Friends, neighbors, coworkers, or community members can fill that gap. A few ways to find supportive contacts include:

1. **Joining community groups**: These might be hobby clubs, volunteer groups, or local centers where people gather for activities (like crafts, gardening, or sports).
2. **Attending support groups for trauma survivors**: A group led by a counselor can let you meet others who have faced PTSD. Hearing similar stories can lower the feeling of being alone.
3. **Online communities**: If leaving the house is hard or if you live far from large towns, online forums or social media groups (moderated by mental health professionals or nonprofits) can offer understanding and advice.
4. **Faith or spiritual communities**: If you follow a certain belief, a local place of worship might have gatherings or study groups where you can meet kind people.

Not every group will be a perfect fit. Some people may not understand what you have been through. Still, finding at least one group or community where you feel safe can open doors for new, helpful friendships.

5. Communication Basics

Talking to others can feel stressful if you are used to holding pain inside. But good communication builds trust and keeps connections strong. Here are some basic tips:

1. **Use "I" statements**: Instead of saying, "You never help me," try "I feel overwhelmed and need some help." This reduces blame and opens space for dialogue.

2. **Listen carefully**: Give the other person time to speak without jumping in. Try to understand their view before sharing your thoughts.
3. **Speak honestly but gently**: Share how you feel, but in a calm tone. If you are angry, take a few deep breaths before talking so you do not lash out.
4. **Set limits**: If certain subjects are too painful right now, let the other person know. You might say, "I'm not ready to talk about that event. Could we focus on something else?"

Effective communication can help you form deeper bonds because others see what you need, and you see how they can help you.

6. Helping Others Support You

Sometimes people want to help but are unsure what to do. Here are a few ideas you can suggest:

1. **Be present**: Ask them to offer quiet support. Maybe they can come over and sit with you if you are having a rough day.
2. **Offer small favors**: A friend or relative can help by cooking a meal, driving you to an appointment, or making some phone calls if you feel overwhelmed.
3. **Respect your space**: If you need to be alone, they should try to understand and not take it personally. Tell them how you will let them know when you are okay to talk again.
4. **Send simple check-ins**: A short message or phone call asking, "How are you doing today?" can remind you that you are not alone.

Being clear about how others can help can reduce their confusion. It also keeps you from feeling frustrated if their attempts to help are off track.

7. Peer Support and Buddy Systems

Some people find it helpful to form a "buddy system" with another person who has gone through trauma. In a buddy system:

1. **You check on each other** regularly, maybe once a week by phone, message, or meeting up.

2. **You agree to listen** without judgment when one of you is distressed.
3. **You share coping methods** that work.
4. **You celebrate steps forward** (for example, if your buddy managed to go shopping without panic for the first time in a long time).

4. **You give simple praise for steps forward** (for example, if your buddy managed to go shopping without panic for the first time in a long time).

This type of peer support is not therapy, but it can be a comforting supplement to therapy. Make sure both parties respect each other's limits. If one of you needs professional help, encourage that instead of trying to handle severe stress on your own.

---

8. Social Media and Online Communities

In today's world, many people use the internet to connect. Online communities can be great if they offer:

1. **Moderation**: Look for groups with clear rules about respectful behavior.
2. **Anonymity**: You can sometimes share feelings without revealing personal details.
3. **Encouraging members**: A helpful community can share ideas, coping tricks, and empathy.

However, be cautious. Some online spaces might have bullying or fake information. If scrolling through posts makes you more anxious or sad, consider leaving that space. Also, be mindful about who you trust with your personal story online.

---

9. Romantic Relationships and Trauma

People with PTSD may notice that their romantic or intimate relationships become complex. Trauma can affect closeness, trust, and communication. If you have a partner, you might:

1. **Explain triggers**: Let them know certain words, sounds, or touches may make you feel unsafe. Ask them to avoid these or use gentle approaches when you seem triggered.
2. **Share what helps you**: Do you need a hug, or do you need space? Everyone is different. Clear guidance helps your partner support you.
3. **Attend counseling together**: Some couples find that seeing a therapist together helps them talk in a safe setting.
4. **Manage guilt**: You might feel guilty if you cannot be as affectionate or relaxed as before. Remember that PTSD is not your fault, and healing takes time.

It is also possible that your partner might not offer good support or might be abusive. If that is the case, focus on your safety first. Building connections that respect and value you is essential.

10. Handling Rejection or Lack of Understanding

Not everyone you approach for support will react well. Some might not believe you, or they might say hurtful things. This can be painful, especially if it comes from a friend or family member. Here are ways to handle rejection:

1. **Acknowledge the sadness**: It is normal to feel upset or disappointed. Let yourself grieve if someone important to you does not give the care you hoped for.
2. **Remind yourself it is not your fault**: Many people do not understand trauma. Their response does not reflect your worth.
3. **Look elsewhere**: If a certain person cannot support you, try other sources—a counselor, a group, or a new friend.
4. **Set new boundaries**: With unhelpful individuals, you might need to reduce contact or avoid certain topics. This protects your emotional health.

Learning who can or cannot support you might take time, but it helps you place your energy in connections that truly help you heal.

11. Supporting Others While Caring for Yourself

You might come across friends or group members who also have PTSD or mental stress. Supporting them can be good, but remember:

1. **Do not take on more than you can handle**: If you are already feeling overwhelmed, politely explain that you need to take care of your own needs first.
2. **Encourage professional help**: It is kind to listen, but if someone is in deep trouble, steer them toward a therapist or crisis line.
3. **Avoid unhealthy "venting" cycles**: Sharing problems can help, but if conversations always spiral into despair without any hope, it might drag you down too. Aim for a balance of listening and supporting.
4. **Keep realistic expectations**: You cannot solve someone else's trauma. You can only offer understanding, share ideas, or direct them to resources.

When supporting others, keep an eye on your own stress level. You need balance to stay well.

---

12. Tips for Meeting New People

Sometimes, after trauma, a person's circle of friends changes. Maybe old friends cannot relate, or you have moved to a new area. Meeting new people can be scary, but it might be worth it. Some suggestions:

1. **Start with shared interests**: If you like reading, try a book discussion group. If you like animals, try volunteering at a pet shelter. Shared interests give you a common topic to start conversations.
2. **Go slowly**: It is okay to join a group and just listen at first. Observe how people interact and decide if you feel comfortable speaking up.
3. **Use safe online platforms**: Some apps or websites focus on connecting people with similar hobbies. Check for reviews or safety guidelines before meeting anyone in person.
4. **Practice conversation openers**: Simple questions like "How long have you been part of this group?" or "What do you enjoy about this hobby?" can break the ice.

Building new friendships takes time, especially when you carry trauma. But the effort can lead to rewarding connections.

---

13. Balancing Social Time and Personal Space

You might swing between wanting to be around others and needing to be alone. Balancing these needs is important:

1. **Schedule downtime**: If you know a gathering is coming up, plan some quiet rest afterward.
2. **Limit big events**: If crowds or noise overwhelm you, think about attending smaller gatherings or going at off-peak hours.
3. **Keep friends informed**: Let close friends know that sometimes you must decline invitations, but it is not personal.
4. **Watch for isolation**: While alone time can help you recharge, too much isolation might worsen sadness or hopelessness. If you notice this pattern, reach out to someone or talk to a professional.

Finding the right mix of social interaction and solitude can help manage stress in daily life.

---

14. Listening Skills for Better Bonds

Strong connections are built not just on sharing your own experiences but also on listening well to others. Good listening involves:

1. **Giving full attention**: Put down your phone or other distractions when a friend is talking.
2. **Using gentle eye contact**: You do not have to stare, but looking at the person shows you care.
3. **Asking questions**: Simple questions like "How did that make you feel?" or "Can you tell me more?" show you are interested.
4. **Avoiding quick fixes**: Sometimes people just need to talk. Suggesting fast solutions might make them feel rushed or unheard.

When you listen well, others feel safe opening up. This skill strengthens connections over time.

---

15. Rebuilding Trust After Betrayal

If your trauma came from someone who was supposed to protect you—like a partner, relative, or authority figure—trust might feel completely shattered. Rebuilding trust can be slow, but it can happen:

1. **Do not rush**: You can go at your own speed when sharing your story or letting someone into your life.
2. **Look for consistency**: Trust grows when a person shows steady, caring behavior over time.
3. **Communicate your fears**: If you worry about being hurt again, talk about it. Let the other person know what helps you feel safer.
4. **Seek support if you feel stuck**: A therapist can guide you through trust-building exercises or help you see signs of healthy vs. unhealthy relationships.

It is okay to be cautious. Over time, you might find people who treat you with respect, proving that trust is still possible.

---

16. The Role of Professional Support in Building Connections

Some people feel more comfortable starting with professional support, such as:

- **Therapists**: They can guide you in learning social skills or help you practice conversations that reduce anxiety.
- **Group therapy**: Led by a counselor, group therapy allows you to share experiences with others in a structured setting. This can lead to friendships after group sessions end.
- **Social workers**: They may connect you to local events, community programs, or volunteer opportunities that help you meet others in a safe environment.

Professional settings can act as a stepping stone to more casual relationships.

---

17. Cultural and Language Factors in Connection

If you belong to a community where mental health is not openly discussed, finding support can be harder. You may need to:

1. **Seek leaders who understand**: Some communities have trusted individuals who act as bridges between mental health support and cultural norms.
2. **Look for language-friendly professionals**: If English (or the main language where you live) is not your first language, find a therapist or group that speaks your language or provides an interpreter.
3. **Adjust communication styles**: Some cultures encourage direct sharing, while others prefer more subtle discussions. Both can work if done with respect.
4. **Stay patient**: Building trust across cultural differences can take time. Keep looking for the right fit.

Your personal background may shape how you form connections. That is okay. You deserve help that respects who you are.

---

18. Protecting Yourself from Harmful Connections

Not all connections are good. Some people might take advantage of your vulnerability or behave in ways that harm your well-being. Stay alert for:

1. **Disrespect or bullying**: If someone mocks your trauma or calls you names, that is not acceptable.
2. **Manipulation**: A friend or partner might guilt-trip you, telling you that you owe them for their support. This is not healthy.
3. **Pushing boundaries**: If you said you do not want to talk about certain details and they keep pressing, consider whether they respect your comfort.
4. **Violence or threats**: If anyone uses force or fear to control you, contact local resources or law enforcement if you feel safe doing so.

Your safety comes first. It is better to have fewer connections than to remain in a harmful one.

Chapter 8: Dealing with Triggers

A trigger is anything that brings back memories of trauma or sparks intense fear, sadness, or anger. Triggers can be very specific—like a sound, smell, place, or photo—or they can be more general, such as being in a crowd or hearing a certain phrase. When PTSD is present, triggers can make a person feel as if they are back in the traumatic event. This can lead to flashbacks, panic attacks, or a strong urge to escape. In this chapter, we will look at ways to figure out your triggers, common reactions they cause, and methods to handle them. Our focus is on practical tips to help you feel more in control when triggers arise.

---

1. Understanding What Triggers Are

A trigger sets off a reaction in the mind and body. After facing trauma, your brain might store deep connections between certain cues and danger. These cues can be:

- **Sights**: Seeing a person who resembles someone involved in your trauma, or noticing a setting that looks like the place it happened.
- **Sounds**: Alarms, loud pops, breaking glass, or even music that was playing during the event.
- **Smells**: A particular fragrance, smoke, or the scent of a certain place.
- **Tastes**: Eating a food that was connected to a traumatic time or location.
- **Feelings**: Emotional states like shame or fear might remind you of the event. Physical feelings (like a racing heartbeat) can also set off memories.

A trigger itself is not dangerous, but the body and mind may respond as if it is. Recognizing triggers is the first step toward managing them.

---

2. Signs You Have Been Triggered

When a trigger occurs, you might notice:

1. **Intense anxiety**: A sudden rush of fear or a panicky feeling.
2. **Racing heart and tense muscles**: You may shake or feel tightness in your chest.

3. **Flashbacks**: Vivid images that make you feel like the trauma is happening again.
4. **Irritability or anger**: Sometimes a trigger can spark sudden rage.
5. **Urge to flee or avoid**: You might leave a place quickly or shut down emotionally.
6. **Confusion or disorientation**: Your mind might freeze, making it hard to speak or think.

These signs can show up within seconds. They can last a few minutes or much longer, depending on the intensity of the trigger and how you respond.

---

3. Mapping Out Your Personal Triggers

We touched on keeping a log in earlier chapters, but here we will focus specifically on mapping out triggers. To do this:

1. **Make a list** of situations or cues that you suspect bring up strong feelings.
2. **Write down how they make you feel** physically, such as sweaty palms or a tight stomach, as well as emotionally (fear, sadness, anger).
3. **Note the intensity level** each time. You might rate triggers on a scale of 1 to 10. This helps you see which ones are the hardest to handle.
4. **Look for patterns**: Do triggers happen at a certain time of day? When you are alone or in a crowd? Around certain people?

This map can guide you in creating a plan. You will learn what to avoid when possible and what you need to handle carefully.

---

4. Planning Ahead for Potential Triggers

Some triggers are avoidable—like not watching certain movies or going to a specific place. But life may require you to face unavoidable ones, such as hearing noises in a city or dealing with scents that pop up unexpectedly. A plan helps you feel prepared:

1. **Use a "go-to" technique**: Have a breathing exercise or grounding method ready to use the moment you sense anxiety rising.

2. **Create a support list**: Write down numbers of trusted people and crisis hotlines you can call if you feel overwhelmed.
3. **Carry calming items**: Keep a small object like a soft cloth, worry stone, or a calming scent that you can smell. This can help you refocus on something neutral.
4. **Practice how to leave or pause**: If you are in a public place, know where the exits, restrooms, or quiet corners are. If you need a break, plan how to step away and calm down.

With a plan, triggers might still startle you, but you will have tools to reduce the intensity.

5. Techniques for Handling Sudden Triggers

When a trigger hits unexpectedly, quick methods can help you stay grounded:

- **5-4-3-2-1 Method**: Look around and silently name five things you see, four you can touch, three you can hear, two you can smell, and one you can taste (or imagine tasting).
- **Slow counting**: Count backward from 10 (or 20) in a steady rhythm. Focus on each number.
- **Deep breathing**: Inhale through your nose for four counts, hold for four, exhale for four, and rest for four. This can slow the heart rate.
- **Self-talk**: Silently say to yourself, "I am safe right now. This is just a reminder, not the real threat."
- **Use your senses**: Run cool water on your hands or hold an ice cube. This can bring your attention to the present.

These methods do not erase the trigger but can lower its power, letting you think more clearly about your next steps.

6. Exposure Methods for Unavoidable Triggers

Sometimes you cannot simply avoid a trigger. For example, driving might be necessary even if it was part of your trauma. Exposure techniques can help:

1. **Gradual exposure**: Tackle the trigger in small steps. If driving is the problem, start by sitting in the car without turning it on. Then take short drives on calm roads before moving to busier ones.

2. **Work with a therapist**: A professional can guide you through slow exposure, ensuring you have coping skills in place.

3. **Notice each improvement**: Each small success—like driving one block—is a sign you are building confidence.
4. **Use rewards**: Treat yourself kindly after facing a trigger. This might be a relaxing bath or listening to your favorite music.

Exposure works best with a plan. You do not want to flood yourself with intense fear all at once, as that can worsen anxiety.

7. Changing Negative Thoughts Linked to Triggers

Triggers are often tied to beliefs like "I am not safe," "I am weak," or "The danger is here right now." Shifting these thoughts can reduce the trigger's effect:

1. **Recognize the thought**: Notice when your mind says something harmful or untrue because of a trigger.
2. **Question it**: Ask yourself, "Is this really true now?" or "Am I mixing past danger with the present?"
3. **Replace it**: Think of a more balanced statement: "That event was real, but it is over. I can take steps to be safe now."
4. **Practice often**: It might feel forced at first, but with repetition, the new thought can settle in.

This approach (often part of Cognitive Behavioral Therapy) can empower you to stop letting triggers take full control of your mind.

8. Grounding Yourself in the Present

Being pulled into the past is a common effect of triggers. Grounding helps you stay in the "now." We have already listed some grounding methods in earlier sections, but here are a few more:

1. **Name objects around you**: Silently say, "I see a table, I see a chair, I see a window." This reminds you that you are in a safe location at the moment.

2. **Listen carefully**: Focus on any soft sounds (like a humming appliance or birds outside). Notice the difference between these normal sounds and any scary memory sounds.
3. **Feel your feet**: Notice the pressure of your feet on the ground. Wiggle your toes if you can. This physical sensation can anchor you in reality.
4. **Check your posture**: Straighten your back if possible and take a slow breath. Shifting your posture can interrupt spiraling thoughts.

Over time, grounding becomes a skill you can use automatically whenever a trigger appears.

---

9. Using Safe Words or Signals

If you have a friend, partner, or family member who supports you, creating a code word or signal can help in trigger moments:

1. **Agree on the word/sign**: Choose a short word or simple gesture that means, "I am feeling triggered."
2. **Explain what you need**: When you use the code, the other person should know what to do—maybe guide you to a quiet room, stay close, or help you find a distraction.
3. **Respect the code**: The supporter must not ignore or joke about it. They should respond quickly and calmly.
4. **Use it sparingly**: Keep this for real trigger moments, so it does not lose importance.

Safe words or signals can reduce the time you spend struggling alone. It also helps loved ones feel useful instead of guessing what you need.

---

10. Handling Nightmares as Triggers

Nightmares can be powerful triggers because they happen when you are most vulnerable—during sleep. Waking up from a bad dream might set off flashbacks or panic. Some tips:

1. **Have a calming routine before bed**: This might include warm tea (decaf), reading something soothing, or gentle stretches.

2. **Keep a low light on**: If total darkness scares you, a dim night light can help you see you are in a safe space when you wake.
3. **Write down the nightmare**: Sometimes putting it on paper can separate it from reality. Then do a calming activity to shift your mind.
4. **Practice going back to sleep**: Deep breathing or a soft sound machine can lull you back to rest if you feel anxious.
5. **Talk to a therapist**: If nightmares are frequent, certain therapies or medications may lower their strength.

Nightmares can shake your sense of safety, but with some planning, you can recover quicker and reduce lost sleep.

---

11. Dealing with Emotional Flooding

Sometimes a trigger causes a flood of emotions—fear, anger, shame—all rushing in at once. It can be overwhelming. To manage emotional flooding:

1. **Pause and name emotions**: "I feel afraid, I feel angry, I feel sad." Labeling them can reduce their power.
2. **Focus on breathing**: Take slow, deliberate breaths to help the body calm.
3. **Find a calmer setting**: If you can, step into a quieter room or go outside where fresh air can soothe you.
4. **Use "why" carefully**: Constantly asking "Why did this happen to me?" can spiral into more sadness. Shift focus to "How can I ground myself right now?"
5. **Engage in a simple task**: Doing something small and easy—like tidying up a desk or coloring in a book—can refocus your mind.

Emotional flooding might still happen from time to time, but you can practice managing it so that it does not consume your entire day.

---

12. Apps and Tools That Help with Triggers

Today, many apps can guide you through breathing exercises, relaxation tips, or quick grounding methods. Some ideas:

- **Calming or mindfulness apps**: They often have short audio clips to walk you through relaxation.

- **Daily mood tracking apps**: They let you note triggers and the intensity of your feelings, helping you see patterns over time.
- **Alarms or reminders**: Setting a gentle reminder on your phone to do a grounding exercise or take a break can reduce stress.
- **White noise or nature sound apps**: If loud sudden noises trigger you, background sounds can mask them.

If you have trouble with technology, ask a friend or relative to help set up these tools. They can be extra layers of support when triggers hit.

---

13. Talking About Triggers with a Therapist

A trained professional can help you:

1. **Spot hidden triggers**: Sometimes a trigger is not obvious. A therapist can help you connect dots, such as how a certain color or time of day might trigger feelings.
2. **Build coping methods**: Therapists can teach skills like "thought stopping," "relaxation training," or "systematic exposure."
3. **Reprocess memories**: Methods like Eye Movement Desensitization and Reprocessing (EMDR) can help your brain handle traumatic memories in a safer way.
4. **Plan for setbacks**: Even with hard work, triggers can flare up. A therapist can prepare you with backup strategies.

Therapy can be a safe place to test new responses to triggers without risking harm to yourself or others.

---

14. Sharing Trigger Details with Loved Ones

It might help to tell trusted individuals about your triggers so they do not accidentally set them off. Some suggestions:

1. **Explain briefly**: You do not have to detail the trauma if it is too painful. A simple statement like, "Loud bangs frighten me because of something that happened in the past," can be enough.

2. **Ask for understanding**: If they know you might panic at fireworks, they can warn you ahead of time or help you find a safe spot.
3. **Let them know how to help**: If you freeze up, do you want them to hold your hand or give you space? Clear instructions can prevent confusion.
4. **Express gratitude**: If they remember your triggers and respect them, let them know you appreciate it. Positive feedback encourages them to continue being supportive.

Sharing trigger info might feel scary, but it can build a safer environment around you.

15. Group Settings and Public Places

Crowded spaces can have many triggers—noise, smells, sudden movements. If you must be in a group setting:

1. **Arrive early**: This lets you pick a seat where you feel safer, like near an exit.
2. **Bring a friend**: Having someone you trust by your side can reduce the fear of unexpected triggers.
3. **Plan an exit**: If things become too much, know how to leave quietly. Drive yourself or have a ride arranged so you are not stuck.
4. **Use distraction tools**: Keep a puzzle game, stress ball, or some music on your phone in case you need a quick mental break.

You can gradually build confidence in public places by taking small steps. Over time, being around others might feel less threatening.

16. Self-Compassion and Triggers

Blaming yourself for having triggers or judging yourself as "weak" only adds more stress. To practice self-compassion:

1. **Recognize triggers as normal**: It is a natural response to trauma. Your brain is trying to protect you, even if it overreacts.
2. **Speak kindly to yourself**: Use phrases like, "I am doing the best I can," or "It is okay to need time to calm down."

3. **Avoid comparing**: You might think others "moved on" faster from similar events. Everyone is unique, and your pace is yours alone.
4. **Give yourself rest**: After facing a tough trigger, allow a bit of quiet time. Rest can help you bounce back.

Being kind to yourself is not about ignoring real dangers. It is about understanding that your emotional wounds need gentle care.

---

17. Handling Triggers in the Workplace or School

You might have triggers that pop up at work or in class, where it is harder to find privacy. Consider these tips:

1. **Plan a quick break**: If you feel panic building, excuse yourself to the restroom or a quiet hallway for a minute.
2. **Have a grounding item in your pocket**: Something small and discreet (like a smooth stone) can help center you without drawing attention.
3. **If you trust a supervisor or teacher**: Share that you sometimes need a brief step-out to manage stress. You can keep details vague if you prefer.
4. **Organize your workspace**: Reduce clutter or keep comforting pictures on your desk to lower baseline stress.

Working or studying with PTSD takes extra effort, but small adjustments can make the day more manageable.

---

18. Recognizing Progress Over Time

Triggers might not vanish, but they can lose intensity. Watch for signs of progress:

1. **Faster recovery**: You still get triggered, but you calm down more quickly than before.
2. **Less severe reactions**: Your heart might race, but you no longer feel the need to run or hide.
3. **Willingness to face triggers**: Maybe you can now watch a certain TV scene or walk in a place that used to cause panic, although you still feel a bit uneasy.

4. **New coping strengths**: You spot a trigger, use a breathing technique, and get back to the present.

Noticing these small gains can remind you that hard work pays off. The goal is not to force yourself to be fearless, but to manage fear in a way that lets you live more freely.

---

19. Knowing When to Seek More Help

If triggers are getting stronger or you feel powerless against them, it might be time for added support:

- **Talk to your therapist**: If you have one, let them know exactly how bad the triggers have become. They may change or intensify your therapy plan.
- **Consider medication**: If panic attacks or flashbacks keep happening, medication might help reduce their severity.
- **Look for trauma-focused specialists**: Some therapists have extra training for complex PTSD or certain types of trauma.
- **Ask about group therapy**: Hearing from others who handle similar triggers can give you new ideas or remind you that you are not alone.

Needing extra help is not a failure. Sometimes triggers grow stronger in response to life changes or stress. You deserve thorough support.

Chapter 9: Staying Calm and Balanced

Sometimes, after living with the stress of PTSD or strong trauma, it can feel like your mind and emotions are in a storm. You might have moments of feeling okay, and then, without warning, you slip into panic or sorrow. Learning how to stay calm and balanced in daily life becomes a key goal. This does not mean you will never feel upset again. Instead, the idea is to develop steady habits that let you return to a more stable emotional state when tension arises. In this chapter, we will talk about what balance means, how to notice when you are off-track, and ways to bring yourself back to a calmer place. We will also address ways to handle changes and make sure you have enough support to keep steady.

1. What Does Calm and Balanced Mean?

Staying calm and balanced does not suggest you must feel positive or peaceful all the time. That is not realistic. Instead, it is about having a baseline sense of stability in your mind and body. When stressful events or triggers show up, you might feel uneasy, but you have the tools to manage those feelings so that they do not take over completely. Being balanced also involves:

- **Having healthy emotional responses**: You can experience a range of emotions—sadness, joy, anger—without getting stuck in them.
- **Feeling steady in your body**: Your heart rate, breathing, and muscle tension are not always at an extreme high or low.
- **Using reliable methods to handle distress**: You know ways to calm yourself if you start to feel out of control.
- **Maintaining awareness**: You notice when tension is building and take action before it becomes overwhelming.

Living in this state helps you make better decisions, enjoy normal activities, and get back on track faster when life throws challenges your way.

2. Why Balance Can Be Hard After Trauma

Trauma can disrupt the body's normal stress systems. You might find your "alarm" response kicks in too often or stays activated longer than it should. Here is why balance might be challenging:

1. **Overactive survival mode**: Your body may remain on guard, ready to fight or flee even when the environment is calm.
2. **Negative thought cycles**: You might struggle with thoughts like "I'm not safe" or "Something bad will happen," which can feed anxious feelings.
3. **Emotional numbness**: In trying to protect yourself from pain, you might push your emotions away so fully that feeling anything becomes difficult, creating an unnatural sense of emptiness.
4. **Ups and downs**: If you spend time feeling on edge, you might later collapse into exhaustion or sadness. These highs and lows can be draining.

None of these are signs of weakness. They are normal responses to trauma. However, they can make it tough to keep a balanced emotional and physical state in daily life.

---

3. Recognizing When You Are Out of Balance

It helps to learn personal clues that indicate you are off-center. These vary from person to person, but common signs include:

- **Trouble sleeping**: Insomnia or waking often during the night.
- **Irritability**: Feeling easily annoyed by small problems.
- **Physical discomfort**: Frequent headaches, stomachaches, or muscle pain.
- **Restlessness**: Having a hard time relaxing or sitting still, as if you need to constantly move or do something.
- **Avoidance**: Dreading everyday tasks because you feel you do not have the energy or focus.
- **Racing thoughts**: Struggling to slow down your mind, which might jump from one worry to the next.

When you see these warning signs, it is time to use strategies that can help you return to a calmer, more balanced feeling. The sooner you notice, the easier it can be to manage.

---

4. The Role of Routines in Maintaining Balance

Having routines can help the body and mind know what to expect. This does not mean creating a strict schedule down to every minute. Instead, you might:

1. **Set regular sleep times**: Going to bed and getting up around the same hour helps your internal clock and reduces chaotic sleep patterns.
2. **Have planned meal times**: Eating around the same times can prevent drops in blood sugar that could lead to mood swings.
3. **Include small breaks**: A short pause to breathe or stretch every couple of hours can lower tension before it builds up.
4. **Designate calming activities**: Whether it is listening to gentle music after work or reading quietly before bed, predictability can calm the stress response.

Routines act like signposts for your body, helping it understand that not every moment is a crisis. Over time, this can make a huge difference in feeling more even and collected.

---

5. Body Awareness and Staying Grounded

One reason trauma can throw you off balance is that it disconnects you from bodily sensations. You might ignore signals like tightening muscles or a quickening heart. Reconnecting with your body can be a powerful way to stay calm:

- **Check in with your body**: Several times a day, pause and notice how you feel physically. Are your shoulders high? Is your jaw clenched?
- **Practice simple relaxation**: If you find tension, you might take a few slow breaths or gently roll your shoulders to release tightness.
- **Use mindful movement**: Activities like gentle stretching, walking, or slow-paced exercises can help you become aware of how your body feels in motion.
- **Notice temperature**: Feeling whether you are too hot, too cold, or just right can bring your focus back to the present.

By paying attention to these signals, you can respond earlier to rising stress and guide yourself back toward calm.

---

6. Emotional Regulation Techniques

Balancing your emotions after trauma involves learning to calm yourself when sadness, anger, or fear surfaces. Here are some methods:

1. **Label your emotion**: Name what you are feeling (e.g., sadness, worry, or frustration). This step alone can reduce the emotion's power.
2. **Step back and observe**: Imagine your emotion as a wave passing by. You watch it rather than let it sweep you away.
3. **Use safe outlets**: If you are angry, you might write about it or squeeze a stress ball. If you are sad, you might allow yourself a gentle cry or share your feelings with a trusted friend.
4. **Limit negative self-talk**: Telling yourself "I shouldn't feel this way" can add shame. Instead, accept that emotions are normal responses.
5. **Shift focus when needed**: After acknowledging the emotion, you may choose a calming action to move forward, such as looking at a soothing photo or smelling a pleasant scent.

These techniques help you handle emotional waves without ignoring them or being completely overwhelmed.

---

7. Balancing Busy Times and Rest

Living with PTSD can make daily tasks feel extra draining. Balancing active times with enough rest is crucial:

- **Pace your day**: If you know certain tasks or events will be stressful, try not to schedule too many of them back to back.
- **Plan recovery periods**: After something demanding—like a work meeting or a social gathering—set aside quiet time.
- **Watch for burnout**: If you feel mentally or physically wiped out, it might mean you have been pushing too hard. This is a signal to slow down.
- **Protect your weekends or off days**: Avoid filling them with more obligations than necessary. Let yourself recharge.

It is easy to feel guilty if you think you are not doing "enough." However, taking breaks can actually help you do tasks more effectively and without the added risk of emotional overload.

---

8. Simple Environment Changes

Where you spend your time can also affect your ability to stay calm:

1. **Declutter**: A messy space can increase stress. Try small steps, like clearing a desk or table.
2. **Consider lighting**: Harsh or flickering lights can raise tension. Softer lighting or using natural light might help.
3. **Add calming elements**: This could be a soft blanket, a gentle scent, or a houseplant.
4. **Minimize loud noises**: If possible, use earplugs or noise-cancelling headphones in busy environments.

These small tweaks can turn your home or workspace into a calmer environment that supports emotional balance.

---

9. Reassessing Personal Boundaries

Staying balanced often requires healthy boundaries. If you are doing too much for others or ignoring your own limits, stress can pile up. Some tips:

- **Learn to say "no"**: Politely decline requests that overwhelm you. You do not need to offer lengthy explanations. A simple, "I can't do that right now" can be enough.
- **Plan for alone time**: If you recharge best on your own, make sure to protect some quiet hours.
- **Limit draining relationships**: If certain people only bring drama or leave you feeling unsafe, consider reducing contact or seeking professional advice on how to manage these ties.
- **Share your needs**: If you live with others, let them know that certain times or places are set aside for your relaxation so they respect your space.

Boundaries can feel uncomfortable at first, especially if you are used to pleasing others. Yet they are a key part of preventing overwhelm and keeping life balanced.

---

10. Handling Quick Surges of Stress

Even if you do everything "right," unexpected stress can burst into your day—a tough phone call, a sudden reminder of trauma, or an urgent responsibility. Here are ways to regain calm fast:

1. **Quick body scan**: Pause, close your eyes if you can, and notice where tension is located (head, neck, shoulders, stomach). Release it using slow exhales.
2. **Use a short phrase**: Something like, "I can handle this," or "One step at a time."
3. **Drink water**: Sipping water can slow your breathing and shift your focus.
4. **Temporarily step away**: If possible, take a brief walk or move to a quieter area.

Training yourself to manage sudden stress in the moment will reinforce a steady baseline of calm.

---

11. Balancing Connections with Personal Needs

In Chapter 7, we focused on building helpful connections. Here, let us emphasize how those relationships affect balance:

- **Enjoy positive contact**: When you feel emotionally stable, spend time with friends or family. These moments can refuel you socially.
- **Set a friend's boundary**: If someone is leaning on you heavily, let them know if it becomes too much. Compassion includes caring for yourself.
- **Take short check-in breaks**: A supportive phone call or text exchange can remind you that you are not alone, but do not let it consume you if you need rest.
- **Alternate activities**: If you had a long talk about heavy topics, do something lighter afterward to prevent emotional overload.

Good connections boost calm, but you must also watch that you do not lose track of your own wellness by focusing only on other people's needs.

---

12. Building Physical Strength and Balance

Balance is not only mental or emotional; it can also be physical. While intense workouts might be stressful for some people, gentle physical activities can support overall calm:

1. **Try light stretching routines**: A few moves in the morning or evening can reduce muscle tightness that feeds anxiety.
2. **Explore low-impact exercise**: Activities like walking, mild aerobics, or using a stationary bike can improve circulation and lower stress hormones.
3. **Stay hydrated**: Dehydration can make you feel tired and irritable.
4. **Breathe well during exercise**: Focus on smooth, steady breaths. This helps the body learn how to stay calm even when moving.

Building physical strength in a gentle way can raise your overall resilience. You might notice you have more energy and fewer aches, which supports a steady frame of mind.

---

13. Creative and Relaxing Outlets

When thinking about balance, do not forget the value of restful and creative outlets:

- **Gentle art projects**: Coloring, sketching, or painting in a relaxed manner can help you unwind without too much mental strain.
- **Soothing music**: Playing soft music in the background can calm the atmosphere in your home.
- **Easy reading**: Choose books or articles that do not provoke strong negative emotions, focusing instead on topics that soothe or gently inspire you.
- **Nature time**: If you can visit a park, garden. or natural spot, even for a short period, it can refresh your mind.

None of these have to be grand hobbies. Even 15 minutes a day of an enjoyable activity can help keep your stress in check.

---

14. Mindful Journaling for Balance

Writing down thoughts is a practice that can foster emotional steadiness:

1. **Clear your head**: Putting worries or confusing feelings on paper can stop them from swirling in your mind.

2. **Spot patterns**: Over time, reading past entries may show certain triggers or repeated issues.
3. **List calming successes**: Write about moments when you handled stress well. This helps you see your own progress.
4. **Keep it simple**: You do not need fancy words—short sentences or bullet points can work.

Journaling can be done daily or whenever you feel tension rising. It is a private place to express feelings and find a bit of relief.

---

15. Accepting Imperfection

Staying calm and balanced does not mean you will do everything perfectly. Some days, despite your best efforts, you may feel anxious or overwhelmed. In these moments:

- **Give yourself grace**: Rather than scolding yourself, remind yourself that healing is a gradual process.
- **Look for small victories**: Maybe you managed to pause and breathe before anger took over. That is still a win.
- **Reach out if needed**: Call a friend or talk to a professional. Sometimes an outside voice helps you see the bigger picture.
- **Try again tomorrow**: Each day is a chance to use or refine your methods.

Part of true balance is knowing that dips happen. Responding kindly to yourself when you stumble can help you rise again more quickly.

---

16. Balancing Technology Use

Technology can be both helpful and overwhelming. Social media, news feeds, and notifications might add stress. Consider:

- **Setting time limits**: Decide how much time you want to spend scrolling social media. Use app timers if needed.
- **Turning off alerts**: Constant pings can keep you on edge. Turn off non-urgent notifications.

- **Choosing content wisely**: Follow pages that uplift or inform gently rather than ones that spread fear or anger.
- **Taking device-free moments**: Try a couple of hours each day without checking your phone or computer, letting your mind breathe.

Technology can help you stay connected, but balance is crucial. Overuse can crowd your mind with more tension than it can handle.

---

17. Dealing with Unexpected Setbacks

Even when working hard to maintain calm, life can bring sudden disappointments—loss of a job, a health scare, or a conflict with someone close. Facing setbacks without losing balance is tough but not impossible:

1. **First, stabilize**: Use quick calming tools—breathing, stepping away—to prevent the shock from escalating.
2. **Gather facts**: Try not to let fear or guesswork drive you. Get clear information about the problem.
3. **Ask for help**: Whether from a professional, a trusted friend, or a helpline. This can keep you from feeling alone in the crisis.
4. **Plan small steps**: Big problems can be overwhelming. Break them into smaller tasks.
5. **Monitor emotional health**: If you feel yourself slipping into negative habits (like oversleeping or substance misuse), act quickly by contacting a support person or therapist.

Setbacks do not mean you have failed at staying balanced. They are part of life. With planning and support, you can weather them while preserving a sense of inner steadiness.

---

18. Tracking Progress to Stay Motivated

When dealing with PTSD, progress might feel slow, and you may forget how far you have come. A simple tracking system can help:

- **Daily or weekly check-ins**: Give yourself a quick score for how calm or balanced you felt.

- **Notice positive changes**: Maybe you are sleeping better, or you recovered faster from a stressful event than before.
- **Compare mindfully**: Look at entries from weeks or months past to see improvements in mood or energy.
- **Share with a counselor**: If you are in therapy, your notes can guide discussions and show areas of growth.

Measuring progress can motivate you to continue practicing the methods that help you remain calm.

---

19. When to Seek Extra Support

Sometimes, even with good habits, staying calm and balanced feels very hard. Signs you might need extra help include:

- **Increased panic attacks**
- **Severe trouble sleeping** that impacts daily function
- **Feelings of hopelessness** or thoughts of self-harm
- **Withdrawal from people or activities you usually like**
- **Substance misuse** (using alcohol or drugs to numb stress)

If any of these are happening, talk to a professional. Adjusting therapy approaches or adding more frequent counseling can keep you from sliding deeper into distress. There is no shame in needing additional support.

Chapter 10: Self-Care and Good Routines

You may have heard the term "self-care" in many places, but it can be confusing to know what it really means. After dealing with trauma, taking care of yourself becomes especially vital because it helps rebuild trust in your own body and mind. Good routines are part of self-care. They create a dependable rhythm in life and offer a sense of control. In this chapter, we will explore what self-care can look like for someone living with PTSD or trauma-related stress. We will also examine the importance of daily habits that protect and nurture your well-being.

---

1. Defining Self-Care

Self-care refers to actions and choices you make to look after your physical, emotional, and mental health. It is not about pampering yourself all day or ignoring life's responsibilities. Instead, self-care is:

- **Listening to your body and mind**: Noticing signals of tiredness, hunger, or emotional strain and responding in a helpful way.
- **Respecting your limits**: Knowing when you have done enough for the day and giving yourself permission to rest.
- **Being proactive**: Setting up routines that keep stress in check, rather than waiting for problems to escalate.
- **Showing yourself kindness**: Treating yourself as you would treat a loved one who is struggling—offering support and understanding instead of harsh criticism.

Self-care is a basic need, especially for those managing PTSD. When you face trauma, your system can become drained. Taking time to refill your emotional and physical energy is not selfish—it is necessary.

---

2. Barriers to Self-Care

Even though self-care is important, many people find it hard to practice:

1. **Feeling undeserving**: Trauma can lead to low self-esteem. You might feel you do not deserve care or rest.

2. **Guilt about taking time**: You may worry that focusing on yourself leaves others without help or that you seem "lazy."
3. **Lack of ideas**: If you have never learned healthy self-care habits, you might not know where to begin.
4. **Overlapping crises**: Sometimes life pressures—like financial struggles or caring for family—can seem too urgent to allow for self-care.
5. **Difficulty breaking habits**: If you are used to ignoring your needs or using negative coping methods, making changes can be tough.

Recognizing these barriers is the first step to overcoming them. With awareness, you can challenge thoughts or situations that block your ability to look after yourself.

---

3. Physical Self-Care

Trauma can affect your body in many ways, so caring for your physical health is essential:

- **Regular check-ups**: See a healthcare provider for routine appointments, even if you feel generally okay. This ensures any concerns are caught early.
- **Nutrition**: You do not need a perfect diet, but aim for balanced meals with enough protein, fruits, vegetables, and whole grains. Avoid skipping meals, as hunger can worsen mood swings.
- **Hydration**: Drinking enough water helps with energy and focus. Dehydration can add to anxiety or headaches.
- **Rest**: Aim for consistent sleep. If nightmares trouble you, consider gentle bedtime rituals like reading something light or doing soft stretches before turning out the lights.
- **Movement**: Light exercise or daily walks can reduce tension. Even brief activity supports better overall physical health.

Caring for your body is not about strict rules or unreachable goals. It is about respecting the body that has carried you through hard times and giving it what it needs to heal.

---

4. Emotional Self-Care

Emotions tied to PTSD can be overwhelming, so finding ways to manage them is a core part of self-care:

1. **Naming your feelings**: If you feel a rush of anger or sadness, telling yourself "I am angry" or "I am sad" can bring clarity.
2. **Allowing safe expression**: You might cry, talk to someone, or write. Bottling emotions up can add more stress.
3. **Practicing calming methods**: Deep breathing or grounding exercises can help when emotions spike.
4. **Seeking help**: If emotional distress is too strong to handle alone, it is okay to reach out to a therapist or a close friend.
5. **Avoiding constant self-criticism**: Pay attention when your thoughts turn harshly against yourself. Consider what you would say to a friend in your situation and apply that kindness to yourself.

Emotional self-care is not about pushing away negative feelings. It is about giving yourself the space and support to handle them without becoming lost in them.

---

5. Mental Self-Care

Trauma can fill your mind with unhelpful thoughts, including blame and doubt. Taking care of your mental world involves:

- **Challenging negative beliefs**: Ask, "Is this fact or fear?" when harmful thoughts arise.
- **Setting a mental boundary**: Limit how long you dwell on a problem before you take a break or do something else.
- **Expanding positive input**: Whether it is reading a book that uplifts you, watching a gentle show, or spending time on a hobby, filling your mind with something that soothes or inspires can help.
- **Learning new skills**: Sometimes building knowledge—like taking a free online course—can enhance self-esteem and provide a positive focus.
- **Relaxing your mind**: Short mindfulness sessions or even simple daydreaming about a calm place can ease mental stress.

In caring for your mental side, you create a more resilient outlook that can stand up against the stress of trauma-related thoughts.

6. Social Self-Care

Having a network of supportive people is part of self-care. Connections can keep you from feeling alone in your struggles. To build social self-care:

1. **Choose safe company**: Spend time with people who accept your feelings, respect your boundaries, and show genuine kindness.
2. **Set healthy limits**: Even good relationships can become draining if you overextend. Let others know when you need time alone.
3. **Join supportive groups**: Whether in person or online, groups for trauma survivors, or just interest-based communities, can offer understanding and fresh perspectives.
4. **Offer and receive help**: Balancing your role in relationships means sometimes supporting others but also being open to asking for help when you need it.

You do not need a huge circle of friends. Even a few quality connections can be enough to provide the sense of comfort and safety that aids your healing.

7. Designing Daily Routines

Good routines are a way to weave self-care into every day. Routines do not have to be rigid, but they can be:

- **Morning routine**: Waking at a reasonable hour, having a light breakfast, and maybe doing a quick stretch.
- **Midday check-in**: Taking a short walk or stepping away from work for five minutes to breathe and refocus.
- **Evening wind-down**: Setting aside screens for at least 30 minutes before bed, maybe reading or listening to gentle music.
- **Weekend or off-day habits**: Planning one fun activity, like visiting a park or watching a favorite show, and giving yourself permission to rest.

The goal is to create a flow to your day that supports your body's natural rhythms and keeps stress from piling up.

8. Meal Planning and Nutrition Routines

Food has a direct impact on mood and energy levels. Making small changes can help stabilize your body and mind:

1. **Plan simple meals**: You do not need complicated recipes. Choose a protein (chicken, beans, fish), a vegetable, and a carbohydrate (rice, bread, potatoes).
2. **Prep ahead**: If cooking each day is stressful, make extra portions and freeze them.
3. **Mindful eating**: Try to eat without watching TV or looking at your phone. Notice flavors and textures. This can calm your mind while you eat.
4. **Balance treats**: Sweets or comfort foods are fine in moderation, but relying on them for every meal can lead to unstable energy and mood swings.

Nutrition is not about perfection; it is about giving your body steady fuel so you can handle PTSD symptoms more effectively.

---

9. The Importance of Rest and Sleep

Trauma can disturb sleep patterns, leading to nightmares or difficulty settling. Yet good rest is key to healing:

- **Keep a bedtime schedule**: Choose a consistent lights-out time.
- **Make your bedroom soothing**: Dim lights, reduce clutter, and set a comfortable temperature.
- **Avoid heavy meals or too much liquid right before bed**: This can disrupt sleep with indigestion or frequent bathroom trips.
- **Write down worries**: If your mind races when you lie down, jot down pressing thoughts in a notebook. This can help you put them aside until morning.
- **Relaxing routine**: Gentle stretching, listening to calming sounds, or reading a calm book can signal your body that it is time for rest.

Good sleep routines can lower anxiety levels and improve your ability to cope with daily stressors.

---

10. Personal Hygiene and Small Rituals

Daily self-care also includes hygiene and small acts that keep you feeling fresh and present:

1. **Regular showers or baths**: Warm water can soothe tight muscles and clear away mental cobwebs.
2. **Brushing teeth or hair**: Doing these tasks mindfully can ground you. Focus on the sensations as you brush.
3. **Using pleasant scents**: A lightly scented lotion or soap can offer a sensory lift without overwhelming you (unless strong smells are triggers).
4. **Dressing comfortably**: Choose clothes that make you feel at ease in your own skin.

These basic tasks, done with attention, can serve as anchors throughout the day, reminding you that caring for yourself is important.

---

11. Structuring Safe Leisure Time

Having time to unwind is part of a balanced routine. Leisure does not have to be fancy or costly:

- **Engage in playful activities**: Try a puzzle, a lighthearted video game, or a simple craft.
- **Explore hobbies**: If you enjoy drawing or playing a musical instrument, set aside time for it.
- **Enjoy nature**: A short walk or sitting in the sun can ease tension.
- **Write letters or emails**: Reaching out to friends or relatives can be a soothing way to connect.

Leisure time can recharge you, helping you face challenges with fresh energy and mental clarity.

---

12. Spiritual or Reflective Routines (If Meaningful to You)

For some individuals, spirituality or quiet reflection is part of self-care:

- **Prayer or meditation**: A few minutes spent in quiet reflection can calm the mind.
- **Reading spiritual or philosophical texts**: This might provide comfort or new perspectives.
- **Reflective walks**: Combining gentle movement with open reflection on feelings or hopes.
- **Gratitude notes**: Listing things you are thankful for (big or small) can shift focus away from constant worry.

Not everyone finds meaning in these practices, and that is okay. If they do resonate with you, they can become part of a powerful self-care routine.

---

13. Tracking Your Self-Care Efforts

If you find it hard to stay motivated, consider tracking your self-care:

1. **Use a habit calendar**: Mark days you completed your chosen self-care tasks (such as going for a walk or writing in a journal).
2. **Make a short checklist**: Ticking off items like "ate a balanced meal," "did a breathing exercise," or "talked to a friend" can provide a sense of completion.
3. **Reflect on benefits**: Write down if you noticed better sleep, less anxiety, or improved mood.
4. **Adjust as needed**: If a routine feels like too much, simplify it. If it feels too easy, add a small challenge.

Tracking is not about being perfect; it is about seeing your efforts and how they affect your well-being.

---

14. Overcoming Resistance to Self-Care

You may notice an internal voice that says self-care is a waste of time, especially if you have a long list of obligations. Here are ways to handle that resistance:

1. **Start with small actions**: Even five minutes of deep breathing or a quick stretch can have a positive effect.

2. **Schedule it**: Put self-care activities on your calendar just like you would a work meeting.
3. **Remind yourself of the benefits**: Think about how even a little care can reduce anxiety, help you focus, or lift your mood.
4. **Seek accountability**: Tell a friend, therapist, or support group about your self-care goal so they can cheer you on or check in with you.

Resistance is normal, but it does not have to stop you. Over time, self-care can become a welcome habit.

---

15. Adjusting Self-Care for Different Life Seasons

Life is always changing. Some periods are busier or more stressful than others. Adjust your self-care to fit current needs:

- **During high stress**: You might need more rest, simpler routines, and quick ways to de-stress.
- **When things are calmer**: You can explore deeper hobbies or take on new wellness challenges.
- **After a setback**: Focus on gentle basics like sleep, light meals, and safe activities before adding bigger tasks.
- **While healing physically**: If you are recovering from an illness or injury, your self-care might center on rest and gentle movement approved by your doctor.

Flexibility keeps self-care useful rather than forcing you to follow routines that no longer suit your situation.

---

16. Staying Consistent

Consistency is where many people struggle. They start a self-care plan but stop after a week. To stay consistent:

1. **Pick realistic activities**: If you hate running, do not plan a daily jog. Choose something you find bearable or mildly pleasant.
2. **Link to existing habits**: For instance, stretch for a few minutes after brushing your teeth each morning.

3. **Set gentle reminders**: Phone alarms or sticky notes can prompt you until the habit forms.
4. **Forgive slip-ups**: If you skip a day, just resume the next one without scolding yourself.

Consistency matters more than intensity. Regular small actions often lead to big improvements in well-being over time.

---

17. Signs That Self-Care Is Working

You might wonder, "How will I know if my efforts are helping?" Possible signs include:

- **Steadier mood**: You might not feel amazing all day, but you notice fewer big emotional swings.
- **Improved energy**: You do not tire as quickly or can handle tasks with less frustration.
- **Better sleep**: Falling asleep more easily or waking up feeling somewhat more rested.
- **Lower anxiety**: Triggers might still arise, but you handle them with more calm or recover faster.
- **Feeling kinder toward yourself**: You notice less harsh self-talk and more gentle thoughts.

Keep in mind that progress may be gradual. Small changes, tracked over weeks or months, can add up to a notable shift in how you feel day to day.

---

18. Combining Self-Care with Therapy

If you are in therapy or counseling for PTSD, self-care routines can support the work you do in sessions:

1. **Share your routines**: Let your therapist know what self-care activities you are trying. They might have extra suggestions.
2. **Use therapy insights**: If you learn a coping skill in therapy, weave it into your daily plan.

3. **Monitor therapy impact**: Good self-care can lessen stress, so you may be more open and engaged in therapy discussions.
4. **Ask for feedback**: A therapist can help you fine-tune your routine so it complements your treatment goals.

Self-care and therapy often boost each other, leading to stronger overall healing.

---

19. Involving Others in Your Self-Care

You do not have to do self-care alone. Including people you trust can deepen the benefits:

- **Family or friends**: Invite a friend to join you on a walk or let a family member know you are trying to cook healthier meals so they can help.
- **Support groups**: Share tips on self-care routines with peers who understand trauma.
- **Online communities**: If in-person support is limited, you might find groups that discuss healthy habits or do daily check-ins for motivation.
- **Professional coaches**: While not always needed, some people find that life coaches or wellness coaches can provide structure and encouragement.

Involving others can make self-care feel less like an isolated task and more like a shared effort, though it is still fine to keep certain parts of your routine private.

Chapter 11: Using Coping Skills

Finding ways to cope when you have Post-Traumatic Stress Disorder (PTSD) or other trauma-related stress can help you feel more stable. Coping skills give you methods to handle triggers, manage difficult emotions, and work through problems that arise. These skills do not take away the fact that you experienced something distressing. Instead, they reduce how much that experience interrupts your current life. Many people discover that with practice, coping skills become a sort of toolkit. You can pull out whichever tool you need in a given moment. This chapter will look at how to pick and use coping methods that match your personal needs. We will also discuss how to keep these skills fresh and adapt them to different situations.

1. What Are Coping Skills?

Coping skills are actions or ideas that help you deal with challenging thoughts, feelings, or memories. Instead of staying stuck in panic or sadness, you use these methods to find relief or to reduce emotional intensity. There are many types of coping skills, such as:

1. **Relaxation methods**: Simple breathing exercises, muscle relaxation, or grounding.
2. **Cognitive skills**: Challenging negative thoughts and replacing them with balanced thinking.
3. **Physical actions**: Taking a brief walk, doing gentle stretches, or using a stress ball.
4. **Distraction tactics**: Listening to soft music, doodling, or focusing on a puzzle.
5. **Social approaches**: Talking to a trusted friend, contacting a support hotline, or joining a peer group.

Each of these can be shaped to suit your preferences. Some people prefer calm, quiet coping strategies, while others find more active methods help them release energy.

2. Why Coping Skills Matter for Trauma Survivors

After trauma, your mind and body can switch into an alarm mode too easily. You might feel anxious or on guard without warning. Coping skills help bridge the gap between feeling overwhelmed and regaining calm. Here are some reasons why they are especially important:

1. **Reducing panic**: Tools like deep breathing or grounding can lower your heart rate and bring your mind back to the present.
2. **Handling triggers**: When you sense a trigger, having a go-to coping skill can prevent a full-blown flashback or meltdown.
3. **Managing relationships**: If anger or irritation flares up, coping skills let you pause and respond more calmly.
4. **Building self-trust**: Knowing you can soothe yourself fosters confidence. You do not feel so powerless against stress.
5. **Supporting therapy**: If you are in counseling, coping methods extend what you learn there into everyday life.

For many people, these tools allow them to live more fully, even while still working through the effects of trauma.

---

3. Creating a Coping Skills List

It can help to write down a list of coping ideas so you remember them when you feel stressed. In a moment of anxiety or panic, it is easy to forget what has helped you in the past. Here is how to begin:

1. **Brainstorm**: Think of activities or thoughts that have ever brought you calm. This could be something as simple as splashing your face with cold water or humming a tune.
2. **Group them**: Arrange them by categories—relaxation, social, physical, and so forth.
3. **Check feasibility**: Make sure each idea is practical. For example, if you only put "walk in nature" but you live somewhere that is unsafe at certain times, you need an indoor alternative.
4. **Keep the list visible**: Post it on the fridge, save it on your phone, or keep it in a small notebook you carry around.

Reviewing your list often can help you pick the right skill in the heat of the moment. You might also ask a counselor, support group or friend for more ideas.

---

4. Relaxation-Focused Coping Skills

Many people find that relaxation is a cornerstone of coping when living with PTSD. Our minds and bodies tense up as if the threat were still present. Relaxation tools can interrupt this tension. Some examples:

4.1 Deep Breathing

- **How it helps**: Breathing slowly gives the brain a signal that you are safe, lowering the production of stress hormones.
- **How to do it**: Inhale through your nose for a count of four, hold for four, exhale through your mouth for four, then rest for four. Repeat several times.

4.2 Progressive Muscle Relaxation

- **How it helps**: By tensing and releasing muscles in different body areas, you recognize the difference between tension and relaxation.
- **How to do it**: Start at your toes—tense them for five seconds, then release. Move up to calves, thighs, stomach, arms, and so on. Focus on the feeling of tightness leaving each zone.

4.3 Visualization

- **How it helps**: Imagining a calming scene can shift your mental focus away from stress.
- **How to do it**: Close your eyes. Picture a peaceful place—maybe a quiet beach or a cozy room. Use all five senses: what do you see, hear, smell, feel, and taste?

These relaxation skills can be practiced at home daily so that they feel more natural when anxiety unexpectedly rises.

---

5. Cognitive Coping Skills

Many trauma survivors have negative thoughts that loop in their minds. You might think, "I am never safe," or "I cannot handle this." Cognitive coping works on shifting these thought patterns to be more balanced:

5.1 Catching the Thought

- **Key step**: Notice when a negative or fearful idea pops up. Often, the first challenge is recognizing the thought instead of letting it control your mood.
- **Example**: You feel anxious about going grocery shopping and think, "Something bad will happen if I leave my home." Pause and label that thought: "I am having a fear-based thought right now."

5.2 Questioning the Thought

- **Reason**: Not every thought is true. Trauma can make the mind assume the worst.
- **Example**: Ask yourself, "Do I have proof that something bad always happens?" or "Am I mixing up a past event with what is happening now?"

5.3 Replacing the Thought

- **Approach**: If your current thought is harmful, choose a balanced one instead.
- **Example**: "I am being careful, and it is daytime. I can handle a short trip to the store. Most trips end up being okay."

This process is central to Cognitive Behavioral Therapy (CBT), but you can use it on your own as well. Over time, challenging negative thoughts often leads to less anxiety.

---

6. Physical Coping Strategies

Since trauma affects both mind and body, coping that involves movement can help release pent-up stress:

1. **Walking or light exercise**: Stepping outside (if it is safe) or moving gently in your home can reduce muscle tension. You do not have to push yourself hard; even a short walk can shift your mood.

2. **Stretching or yoga-inspired poses**: If it is safe for you and does not bring up negative memories, gentle stretches can calm the body.
3. **Using a stress ball**: Squeezing a small ball or rolled-up sock can help channel nervous energy.
4. **Pacing**: Some people find walking back and forth in a safe area helps them manage anxiety.

Try different physical strategies to see which ones leave you feeling calmer or less overwhelmed. Just remember to respect your body's limits, especially if you have injuries.

---

7. Distraction as a Short-Term Coping Skill

Distraction does not solve problems, but it can give you time to cool down. If you are in the middle of a panic or spiral of fear, distraction can bring quick relief:

- **Puzzles or word games**: They demand enough mental focus to steer your thoughts away from distress.
- **Easy crafts**: Coloring, knitting, or small art projects can keep your hands busy and your mind calmer.
- **Light reading**: A short story, comic, or magazine might help. Avoid materials that could spark negative memories.
- **Cleaning a small area**: Some people find tidying a shelf or organizing a drawer helps them regain a sense of control.

Distraction is most useful for immediate relief. Later, you can return to process your feelings more deeply if needed.

---

8. Social and Support-Based Coping

Sometimes, being with people who understand or care about you can help ease distress. Social coping can include:

1. **Talking with a friend**: If you feel safe, share what is on your mind. Even a short text message like, "I am feeling stressed right now," might bring some support.

2. **Calling a crisis line**: If you are alone and overwhelmed, crisis hotlines or text lines can connect you to a caring listener right away.
3. **Joining a support group**: Online or face-to-face groups for trauma survivors may help you pick up new ideas and feel less alone.
4. **Buddy system**: Pair up with someone else who experiences anxiety or PTSD. You can check on each other regularly.

People who support you can remind you that you are not defined by the bad event. They can also share tips if they have found something that works for them.

9. Adapting Coping Skills to Different Situations

Not every coping skill works in every scenario. For instance, if you feel a panic attack coming on at your workplace, it might not be possible to lie on the floor and do a long relaxation routine. Here is how to adapt:

1. **Consider environment**: If you are in public, choose something discreet like slow, steady breathing or a calming word repeated silently.
2. **Consider time**: If you have only a minute, pick a quick approach such as counting backward from 10. If you have 10 minutes, you might do a guided relaxation exercise.
3. **Consider your energy level**: If you are exhausted, an intense workout might be too hard. A gentle stretch or sipping water might be better.

Being flexible helps you keep using coping strategies instead of giving up when the first one you try is not a good match for the moment.

10. Coping with Anger and Irritability

Trauma can sometimes show up as anger rather than fear. You might be easily provoked, snapping at loved ones or feeling a surge of rage at small annoyances. If that happens:

- **Recognize early signs**: Is your jaw clenching? Are you pacing or feeling heat in your chest? Catch anger before it explodes.
- **Pause and breathe**: Even a few seconds of deep breathing can prevent an outburst.

- **Use mental images**: Picture a stop sign in your head. This can remind you to not say or do something hurtful in the moment.
- **Take a break**: If possible, remove yourself from the situation until you calm down.
- **Problem-solve later**: Anger is often masking deeper feelings like fear or shame. When calm, think about what truly triggered you and see if there is a solution.

Learning anger coping skills can save relationships from unnecessary conflict, and it can reduce shame or regret afterward.

---

11. Coping with Sadness or Depression

Trauma can also spark deep sadness. You may feel numb, hopeless, or unmotivated. Coping strategies for sadness often focus on gentle actions:

1. **Easing into activity**: If it seems impossible to do chores or go outside, start with something very small, such as making your bed or taking a short shower.
2. **Soothing environment**: Listening to soft music, lighting a gentle-scented candle, or tidying a corner of your space can lift your mood a bit.
3. **Nature contact**: If you are up to it, stepping into fresh air or looking at greenery can offer a mild boost.
4. **Reaching out**: Depression can make you isolate. Try sending a quick message to someone, even if you do not feel like talking much.
5. **Balanced self-talk**: Remind yourself that sadness does not define you forever. Emotions can change over time.

If sadness is extreme or long-lasting, you might consider professional help, such as counseling or possibly medication.

---

12. Building Emotional Resilience with Coping Skills

Using coping tools consistently can help you build resilience—an ability to recover after a setback. Here is how:

- **Practice daily**: Do not wait until you are in crisis. Use small calming or positive coping methods daily.

- **Reflect on what worked**: After you use a coping method, think about whether it helped. If it did not, adjust.
- **Combine strategies**: For instance, pair deep breathing with a quick phone call to a friend for double the effect.
- **Keep learning**: There are many new techniques out there. If you find your current set of skills becoming stale, ask a therapist or look for reputable resources on new coping ideas.

Little by little, these efforts can make it easier to bounce back from stress. You might still feel fear or sadness, but it will not hold you captive as long.

13. Dealing with Cravings or Urges to Return to Old Habits

Sometimes, a trauma survivor may have used harmful habits like alcohol misuse, smoking, or risky behaviors to cope in the past. If you have an urge to return to those old habits:

1. **Pause**: Notice the urge before acting on it.
2. **Name the urge**: Say, "I feel a pull to drink right now," or "I want to escape."
3. **Check your coping list**: Choose a safer method instead.
4. **Contact support**: If the urge is strong, call or message someone, or go to a support group meeting.
5. **Show compassion**: A relapse or slip does not mean you have failed. It means you need more support or a different approach at that moment.

Replacing harmful habits with healthier coping is a process, but one that can lead to far better long-term well-being.

14. Creating a "Safe Space" at Home

One helpful coping idea is to set up a small area in your home that you associate with calm. It does not have to be big. It could be a corner of a room. In this space, you might have:

- **Soft lighting**: A gentle lamp or twinkle lights instead of harsh overhead bulbs.
- **Comfort items**: Pillows, blankets, or a plush chair.

- **Relaxing scents**: A mild candle or essential oil if you are not triggered by smells.
- **Positive reminders**: Quotes or photos that bring a sense of safety.
- **Coping tools**: Stress ball, coloring book, headphones for music, or a small puzzle.

When you feel stressed, spend a few minutes here using whichever coping method you prefer. Over time, your brain may learn to associate this space with relaxation.

15. Using Written Coping Plans

A coping plan is a bit more detailed than a simple list. It might outline:

1. **Warning signs**: For example, "When I start sweating or shaking" or "When I notice I am snapping at others."
2. **First steps**: "Close my eyes and take three slow breaths."
3. **Secondary actions**: "If still anxious, text my friend or look at a calming picture."
4. **Who to contact**: Names, phone numbers, or hotlines for support.
5. **Safe places to go**: If being in your current location is too overwhelming, note a place you can safely move to, even if it is just another room.

Review your plan at least once a week so it stays fresh in your mind. This clarity can be a lifesaver when panic hits.

16. Coping During Therapy or Counseling Sessions

In therapy sessions, you might address painful memories. Sometimes those discussions can trigger strong emotions. Using coping skills during therapy can help:

- **Communicate with your therapist**: If you start to feel overwhelmed, let them know right away.
- **Use small breaks**: Ask if you can take a short pause to breathe or stretch.
- **Apply grounding**: If a memory is too vivid, focus on an object in the office. Note its shape, color, and texture.

- **Practice with your therapist**: They can teach or rehearse coping skills with you so you become more comfortable using them outside sessions.

Therapy is a great time to try out different methods in a supportive setting. This preparation can make coping easier in daily life.

---

17. Teaching Coping Skills to Children or Family Members

If you have kids or other family members who are also dealing with trauma, you can adapt coping skills for them:

1. **Use simple language**: For a child, call a deep breath a "balloon breath." Encourage them to imagine their belly filling like a balloon.
2. **Make it fun**: Turn grounding into a game: "Name one thing you can see that is red, one thing that is green, and so on."
3. **Lead by example**: If your family sees you practicing a coping technique, they might follow.
4. **Set up family signals**: You could have a family word that means, "I need a calming moment." Everyone then respects a pause.

By sharing coping skills, you build a supportive environment where each person knows how to calm themselves and support others.

---

18. Knowing When to Adjust Your Coping Methods

Coping is not static; what works now might not work forever. Watch for signs you need to switch things up:

- **Less effectiveness**: A method that used to calm you might no longer help. You could feel just as anxious or upset afterward.
- **Lifestyle changes**: If you move or change jobs, some coping ideas might be less practical.
- **New triggers**: Sometimes new stressors or memories appear, calling for different approaches.
- **Physical changes**: If you develop a health condition, you might need gentler methods.

Adjusting coping methods is normal. You can always talk with a therapist or friends who also use coping skills to get fresh ideas.

---

19. Measuring the Success of Your Coping Skills

How do you know a coping skill is truly helping? You might:

1. **Track your mood**: Keep a little record of your stress level (1–10) before and after using a skill. Over time, see if certain methods show a clear drop in stress.
2. **Look for changes in behavior**: Do you feel less need to avoid certain places or less urge to lash out at others?
3. **Notice patterns**: Sometimes it takes repeated use to see a shift. A single time might not be enough.
4. **Ask for outside observations**: A friend or therapist might see that you seem calmer or more willing to face triggers.

Success does not mean you never feel upset. It means you recover faster and cope better when upset happens.

Chapter 12: Facing Flashbacks and Bad Dreams

Flashbacks and bad dreams are among the most unsettling parts of living with PTSD or deep trauma. They can appear without warning, throwing a person into vivid memories or intense nightmares that feel nearly as real as when the event happened. While these episodes can be very frightening, it is possible to lessen their power over you. This chapter explores what flashbacks and bad dreams are, why they happen, and how to manage them using a range of strategies. By understanding how they arise and applying practical approaches, you can gradually weaken their grip on your daily life.

---

1. Understanding Flashbacks

A flashback is a sudden, intense feeling that you are reliving a past traumatic event. It can involve images, sounds, or other senses that mimic the original experience. During a flashback:

- **You might feel detached from the present**: It is as if you have stepped back in time to the traumatic situation.
- **Your body responds as if danger is real**: Heart rate soars, breathing quickens, muscles tense up, and you might sweat or tremble.
- **You might lose sense of where you are**: The environment around you fades, replaced by the memory.

Flashbacks can be brief or last for several minutes. In extreme cases, they may continue until something interrupts them, like a loud noise or a person speaking to you. Some people experience partial flashbacks, where they do not fully lose awareness of the present but still feel overwhelmed by a strong memory.

---

2. Causes and Triggers of Flashbacks

Flashbacks often spring from triggers—reminders that connect to the traumatic event. These can include:

1. **Sensory triggers**: A smell (like smoke), a sound (like fireworks), or a sight (someone wearing a uniform similar to the person who harmed you).

2. **Emotional states**: Feeling helpless, cornered, or betrayed in a current situation might bring up old memories.
3. **Dates or anniversaries**: When the date of the trauma returns, some people notice an increase in flashbacks.
4. **Environments**: Being in a place that resembles where the trauma took place.

Understanding your personal triggers can help you plan ways to handle them or avoid them if possible. But sometimes, flashbacks occur with no clear trigger at all.

---

3. Types of Flashbacks

Not all flashbacks look the same. Some possibilities:

- **Visual flashbacks**: You see images from the trauma as if watching a movie in your mind.
- **Emotional flashbacks**: You might not have a specific image, but you feel the same emotions—fear, shame, panic—just as strongly as before.
- **Body memory flashbacks**: You sense pain or other body sensations linked to the trauma, such as feeling tightness in your chest or tension in your limbs, even if there is no current cause.
- **Combination flashbacks**: Some people experience a blend of visual, emotional, and physical flashbacks.

Recognizing which type you experience can guide you in choosing the best coping skills. For example, if your flashbacks are mostly about physical sensations, grounding that focuses on body awareness might be effective.

---

4. Immediate Grounding for Flashbacks

Grounding is one of the fastest ways to try to exit or reduce a flashback. Here are several immediate methods:

1. **Name the present**: Silently tell yourself, "I am safe right now. I am [your name]. Today is [date]. I am in [location]. The memory is in the past."

2. **Use five senses**: Look around and name five objects, four sounds, three things you can touch, two things you can smell, and one thing you can taste. This approach forces your mind to notice the present environment.
3. **Run cool water over your hands**: The sensation of water can pull you out of the memory loop.
4. **Hold a grounding object**: A small stone, a stress ball, or a piece of fabric can anchor you. Focus on its texture, temperature, and shape.

These quick approaches can help you regain enough control to remember you are not in the original trauma anymore.

---

5. Handling Flashbacks in Public Places

It is scary to have a flashback in a public space, such as a store or a busy street. You might worry about drawing attention or being unable to hide your distress. Some suggestions:

1. **Learn discreet methods**: Breathing exercises or repeating a calming phrase in your mind can be done without anyone else noticing.
2. **Find a quiet corner**: Step into a restroom or a hallway if possible. Take a moment to breathe or do a grounding action.
3. **Carry a coping card**: Write something like, "I am safe. Breathe. This feeling will pass. Call a friend if needed." Glancing at it can help you refocus.
4. **Prepare an exit plan**: If you can, arrange to leave early or have your own transportation so you do not feel trapped.

Even if you cannot stop the flashback fully, these steps can minimize how long it lasts or how intense it becomes.

---

6. What Are Bad Dreams and Nightmares?

Bad dreams and nightmares related to trauma bring distressing themes or images during sleep. While a "bad dream" might be unsettling but less vivid, a "nightmare" often feels very real and frightening. You might wake up with a racing heart, sweating, or shaking. People with PTSD sometimes face recurring nightmares that mirror the traumatic event, such as seeing or hearing the actual scene again. Others have symbolic nightmares that carry the same sense of terror without the exact details.

7. Effects of Bad Dreams on Daily Life

Frequent nightmares can lead to:

- **Poor sleep**: You might struggle to fall asleep or fear going back to sleep after a nightmare, leading to exhaustion.
- **Avoidance behaviors**: You might avoid resting or resist going to bed, fearing the nightmares.
- **Irritability and anxiety**: Lack of sleep can worsen your mood and make you more easily triggered by daytime stress.
- **Daytime flashbacks**: Being tired can lower your ability to cope with triggers. This might cause more daytime flashbacks.

Interrupting the cycle of nightmares is crucial for better overall well-being, since good rest is a key part of healing.

8. Strategies for Lessening Nightmares

While it is not always possible to control your dreams, you can take steps to reduce their frequency or intensity:

1. **Safe bedtime routine**: Spend time winding down with quiet music, soft lighting, or a short relaxation exercise. Avoid violent or upsetting TV shows before bed.
2. **Write down worries**: If anxious thoughts keep popping up, jot them on paper and set them aside. This can help your mind feel more at ease.
3. **Limit caffeine and alcohol**: These can disrupt sleep quality. Even if alcohol makes you fall asleep faster, it can worsen nightmares later in the night.
4. **Relaxation techniques**: Deep breathing or progressive muscle relaxation just before you lie down can calm your body.
5. **Comforting scents or items**: A mild scent you find pleasant (like lavender, if it is not a trigger) or a soft blanket can help associate bedtime with safety.

Even if nightmares still happen sometimes, these steps can lower how strong and frequent they are.

---

9. Imagery Rehearsal for Nightmares

Imagery Rehearsal Therapy (IRT) is a technique sometimes suggested for trauma-related nightmares:

1. **Recall the nightmare**: Identify the main storyline or emotion.
2. **Change the story**: Write a new, less distressing ending or alter the frightening scenes.
3. **Practice the new version**: Spend a few minutes each day quietly picturing the changed dream.
4. **Reinforce safety**: Remind yourself that you have control over how the story plays out in your mind.

For some people, rewriting the nightmare helps reduce how terrifying it feels. If you find this too stressful alone, you might work on it with a therapist.

---

10. Facing Recurrent Themes in Flashbacks or Dreams

Some individuals find that the same elements appear over and over in their flashbacks or nightmares—such as a locked door, a particular face, or a certain type of location. This repetition can be very upsetting. However, it also provides clues:

- **Identify the theme**: Ask yourself, "What is this repeated element? Is it about feeling trapped, guilty, or powerless?"
- **Link to the original event**: Sometimes these themes represent a key part of the trauma.
- **Talk about it in therapy**: Discussing the repeated themes might help you process the underlying fears or guilt.
- **Use coping images**: If a locked door appears, imagine yourself holding the key or finding a safe exit. Practice this in your mind when you are calm.

Recurrent themes suggest your mind is trying to work through the trauma. Addressing them directly can lessen their grip on your flashbacks and dreams.

11. Using Calming Methods After a Flashback or Bad Dream

It is common to feel shaken or disoriented afterward. You might need extra steps to soothe yourself once it ends:

1. **Reorient to the present**: Turn on a light, look at the time, remind yourself of your name and location.
2. **Drink water or have a light snack**: Focusing on an everyday act can help ground you.
3. **Use gentle movement**: Stretch your arms and legs, or stand up and walk around briefly.
4. **Talk to someone if possible**: A short call or text to a friend can reassure you that you are back in a safe reality.

How you handle the aftermath can affect how long it takes to settle your nerves. Having a short plan for "post-flashback" or "post-nightmare" care can speed recovery.

12. Long-Term Approaches to Flashbacks and Nightmares

While immediate coping skills help in the moment, long-term progress may involve deeper work:

- **Trauma-focused therapy**: Methods like Eye Movement Desensitization and Reprocessing (EMDR), Cognitive Processing Therapy, or Prolonged Exposure can reduce the intensity of flashbacks over time.
- **Medication**: Sometimes, doctors prescribe medications that help reduce nightmares or anxiety. This is a personal choice; some people benefit from it, while others prefer therapy alone.
- **Lifestyle changes**: Regular exercise, healthy eating, and enough rest can boost resilience, making flashbacks or nightmares less dominant.
- **Ongoing support**: Continuing to talk with a counselor, peer group, or supportive friend can keep you from feeling isolated in your struggle.

Over months or years, many people see a drop in the intensity or frequency of their flashbacks and nightmares if they stick with a balanced treatment plan.

13. Helping Children with Flashbacks or Nightmares

Children might have trouble describing these experiences, so watch for signs such as screaming at night, bedwetting, or refusing to sleep alone. Tips for helping kids:

1. **Reassurance**: Let them know they are not bad or weak for having scary dreams or memories.
2. **Simple explanations**: "Sometimes our brain replays upsetting events, but it is only a picture in our head. It cannot hurt us now."
3. **Comfort objects**: A soft toy or nightlight can make bedtime feel safer.
4. **Professional help**: If flashbacks or nightmares persist, consider a therapist who specializes in child trauma.

Kids respond well to routines and gentle guidance. They need a safe environment and adult support to handle these fears.

---

14. When to Seek Emergency Help

Flashbacks or nightmares can sometimes push a person to the edge. If you or someone you know:

- **Feels suicidal or self-destructive**
- **Cannot return to reality after a flashback** for a prolonged period
- **Has a severe panic response that does not calm down**
- **Feels the urge to harm others during a flashback**

It is important to reach out for emergency help. Call local emergency services or crisis hotlines. In some areas, you might be able to go to a hospital for urgent psychiatric care. There is nothing weak about asking for immediate assistance when you feel out of control.

---

15. Dealing with Shame or Embarrassment

Flashbacks and nightmares can bring feelings of shame, especially if they happen in front of others. You might worry about appearing "crazy." Remember:

- **Many trauma survivors experience this**: You are not alone or unusual.

- **It is not your fault**: You did not choose to have the trauma, and your body's response is not a character flaw.
- **Educate supportive people**: If possible, explain that you have a condition that sometimes causes these reactions.
- **Learn from slip-ups**: If you reacted in a way that upset someone, you can apologize but also clarify that you were experiencing a flashback.

Over time, understanding that flashbacks and nightmares are part of how some bodies handle trauma can reduce self-blame.

16. Supporting a Partner or Friend Who Has Flashbacks

If you care about someone with PTSD:

1. **Stay calm**: If they have a flashback, speak to them in a gentle, steady voice.
2. **Ask before touching**: They may be startled by sudden contact if they are "back" in the traumatic moment.
3. **Use grounding questions**: "Can you tell me where we are right now?" or "Do you see me here?"
4. **Show patience**: Scolding or trying to force them to "snap out of it" can worsen fear.
5. **Help them debrief**: Afterward, they might need to talk about it or just rest. Let them choose.

Your calm presence can help them feel safer and recover quicker.

17. Keeping a Flashback and Dream Journal

Some people track their flashbacks and nightmares to notice patterns:

- **Record details**: Note date, time, triggers, and how long it lasted.
- **Describe feelings**: What emotions or bodily sensations were strongest?
- **Write coping steps used**: Did they help, or do you want to try something else next time?
- **Review for patterns**: You might find certain triggers that show up often. A therapist can help interpret your notes.

Journaling can feel upsetting at first, so only do this if you have safe ways to handle strong feelings that may arise. However, it can provide clues that lead to better management.

---

18. Building Nighttime Routines for Better Rest

Because nightmares often strike at night, a peaceful bedtime routine can make a difference:

1. **Set a fixed bedtime**: Consistency teaches your body when to wind down.
2. **Avoid screens an hour before bed**: Bright lights and stimulating content can stir up anxious feelings.
3. **Try gentle stretches**: Loosen tight muscles so your body is not holding extra tension.
4. **Use a nightlight if needed**: Darkness can be triggering for some.
5. **Keep comforting items by the bed**: A favorite pillow or blanket, a glass of water, maybe a small note reminding you of a calming thought.

Doing these things every night can help signal your brain that it is time to rest, potentially lowering the chance of nightmares.

Chapter 13: Changing Negative Thoughts

It is common for people who have been through scary or harmful events to see the world and themselves in a negative light. They might think they are "broken," that danger is around every corner, or that no one can be trusted. Over time, these thoughts can become habits in the mind—popping up without any effort, like a well-worn path that is hard to leave. Changing such thoughts takes patience, but it is possible. When you shift the way you look at yourself and your experiences, you can start to feel lighter and more confident. This chapter explores how negative thoughts develop, why they keep hanging on, and how you can gently replace them with more balanced ideas about yourself, other people, and the future.

1. Why Negative Thoughts Show Up

Negative thoughts often begin as a form of self-protection. When someone has faced a harmful event, the mind tries to guard against future harm. This can lead to thoughts like:

- **"I am always in danger."**
- **"I must be on guard all the time."**
- **"If something bad happened once, it will happen again."**

These thoughts may have been useful in the moment of danger, helping you stay alert. But when the crisis ends, the brain can get stuck in this fearful state. You may continue thinking about all the ways you could be hurt or what mistakes you might make next. Such thoughts act like a false alarm, always sounding even when you are relatively safe.

Negative thoughts can also be fueled by guilt or shame. If you went through a scary time, you might blame yourself for not stopping it. Even if you logically know you are not to blame, a deep feeling of shame can tell you otherwise. Over time, your mind might repeat messages like, "I am worthless," or "I should have done more." These messages can feel true, especially if the trauma took place when you were young or if someone else blamed you for what happened.

2. Recognizing Patterns of Negative Thinking

You may be so used to self-blame or fear-based thinking that you do not notice it anymore. A big step is to recognize when your thoughts are unfair or untrue. Here are some common negative patterns:

1. **All-or-nothing thinking**: Seeing the world in extremes. For example, "Nobody cares about me" or "I fail at everything." There is no middle ground.
2. **Overgeneralizing**: Taking one event and assuming it always happens. "I got into one fight with a friend, so I must be a terrible person."
3. **Disqualifying the positive**: Ignoring any good things that happen, focusing only on bad events or what might go wrong.
4. **Mind reading**: Guessing that others are judging or disliking you without real proof.
5. **Blaming yourself unfairly**: Believing you caused something terrible, even if you had little or no control.

When you spot these patterns, do not judge yourself. Simply notice, "Oh, that might be overgeneralizing," or "Maybe I am ignoring the good things." This gentle noticing is an important first step toward change.

---

3. Effects of Negative Thoughts on Daily Life

Negative thoughts do more than cause sadness. They can affect all parts of your day. You might:

- **Avoid opportunities**: If you think you will fail or embarrass yourself, you may never try new things.
- **Feel drained**: Constant fear or guilt leaves little energy for friends, hobbies, or enjoying normal activities.
- **Struggle in relationships**: Thinking "No one can be trusted" may push you to keep distance from people who might otherwise be caring.
- **Develop physical problems**: Ongoing stress from negative thinking can lead to headaches, stomach issues, or trouble sleeping.
- **Get stuck**: Without checking these thoughts, you might replay the same worries or regrets endlessly, never moving forward.

Many people feel discouraged by these effects. That is why it is so important to learn new ways of thinking that are fairer, more flexible, and more in line with reality.

4. The Connection Between Thoughts, Feelings, and Actions

In many forms of therapy, there is a concept called the "thoughts-feelings-actions triangle." It says that each part influences the others:

1. **Thoughts**: What your mind says about a situation.
2. **Feelings**: Emotions that arise because of these thoughts (sadness, anger, fear, hope).
3. **Actions**: How you respond—maybe you withdraw, get angry, or reach out for help.

If your thoughts are very negative, your feelings might be more intense or hopeless. That can lead to actions like isolation or giving up. But when you learn to question your thoughts and see them more clearly, you might find a softer or more balanced perspective. This can ease negative feelings and encourage healthier actions.

5. Catching Negative Thoughts

You cannot replace negative thoughts if you do not notice when they appear. The first skill is "thought catching." This might seem simple, but it takes practice:

- **Keep a small notebook or use a notes app**: When you notice you are feeling down or anxious, write down the thought you are having.
- **Use gentle language**: Instead of saying, "I am so stupid for thinking that way," try, "I notice I just had a thought that says 'I cannot do anything right.'"
- **Mark the situation**: Note what was happening when that thought popped up. Were you at home alone, at work, or talking with a friend? Triggers can help you see patterns.
- **Write how strong the thought felt**: Maybe rate it from 1 (weak) to 10 (overwhelming).

This tracking helps you be aware of common mental habits. You might see that you think "I am not safe" most often when you watch a certain type of movie or when you are around specific people. Awareness is key before you can challenge or change anything.

6. Challenging the Thought

When you spot a negative thought, ask it questions to see if it truly holds up:

1. **Evidence for and against**: Write down facts that support the thought and facts that go against it. For instance, if the thought is "Nobody wants to be my friend," you might list times people have invited you somewhere or shown kindness.
2. **Alternative views**: If your original thought is, "I am worthless," consider other possibilities: "I have flaws, but I also have good qualities" or "I feel worthless right now, but that does not mean I am truly worthless."
3. **What if a friend said this?**: Imagine a close friend shared the same negative statement about themselves. Would you agree with them, or would you remind them of their positive qualities? Often, we are kinder to others than to ourselves.

Keep in mind, challenging a negative thought is not about ignoring real problems. It is about seeing if your inner talk is fair or if it is heavily colored by fear or shame left over from trauma.

7. Replacing with Balanced Thoughts

After questioning a negative thought, you can shape a new thought that feels more accurate. This does not mean you force yourself to be overly positive. Instead, you look for a thought that is true yet less hurtful:

- **Negative Thought**: "I am never going to get better."
- **Balanced Thought**: "Healing takes time, and I have made small signs of progress. I can keep working toward feeling better."
- **Negative Thought**: "I caused the traumatic event."
- **Balanced Thought**: "I had limited control in that situation. I did what I could at the time. The blame belongs to the person or circumstances that caused the harm."

At first, these new thoughts might not feel as natural. However, with repetition, you can weaken the old pathways and create new ones in your brain.

8. Dealing with Persistent Thoughts

Some negative thoughts refuse to let go, even when you try to challenge them. This is often the case with very deep beliefs that formed in response to major trauma, such as childhood abuse or repeated traumatic incidents. In such cases:

1. **Use multiple strategies**: Talk therapy, writing exercises, or even creativity (like drawing your feelings) can help break down stubborn beliefs.
2. **Remind yourself healing is gradual**: Changing thoughts that have been ingrained for years may take steady effort.
3. **Seek professional help**: A counselor or therapist trained in trauma can guide you through techniques like EMDR (Eye Movement Desensitization and Reprocessing) or CBT (Cognitive Behavioral Therapy), which target deep-rooted beliefs.

---

9. Handling Thoughts of Hopelessness or Self-Blame

Trauma survivors sometimes struggle with hopelessness: "Nothing will ever change," or "I can't fix this." They might also feel strong self-blame: "It is all my fault." Here are some ideas for each:

Hopelessness

- **Identify specific worries**: Hopelessness can be vague. If you list specific fears ("I am scared I will never find peace" or "I worry I can't keep a job"), you can tackle them one by one.
- **Look back at past successes**: Even if they seem small, recall times you coped well. This shows you that some good changes are possible.
- **Expand your support**: Talking to others who have come through trauma can spark hope that your situation is not permanently dark.

Self-Blame

- **Consider your control**: Reflect on how much power you truly had during the event. Often, trauma occurs because someone else misused their power or because of forces outside your control.
- **Talk to someone objective**: A therapist or friend can give an outside viewpoint. They might remind you that you were a victim, not the cause.

- **Practice self-forgiveness**: If you blame yourself for not doing something differently, remember you did the best you could with the information and resources you had at that time.

---

10. Building Self-Compassion

Negative thoughts often go hand in hand with harsh self-judgment. Developing compassion for yourself can soften these thoughts. Here are some ways:

1. **Use kind words**: Instead of "I'm so stupid," say "I made a mistake, but I can learn and move on."
2. **Imagine your younger self**: Think of yourself as a child who went through something scary. Would you blame that child, or would you comfort them?
3. **Balance your view**: Recognize that everyone has strengths and weaknesses. You have good traits even if you do not see them right now.
4. **Seek supportive connections**: Spending time with people who treat you well can reinforce the idea that you deserve kindness.

Self-compassion is not about ignoring facts or denying faults. It is about seeing yourself as worthy of patience and understanding, just like anyone else.

---

11. Repetition and Practice

Changing long-held thoughts is like learning a new skill. You need regular practice:

- **Daily check-ins**: Spend a few minutes each morning or evening noting your main thoughts of the day. Gently challenge any negative ones.
- **Use reminders**: Sticky notes on your mirror, positive affirmations in your phone, or a list of balanced thoughts in your wallet can keep you on track.
- **Practice when calm**: It is tough to think clearly if you are very upset. So rehearse new thoughts when you feel okay, so they come to mind faster in stressful moments.
- **Be patient**: Some days you may slip back into old thinking. That is part of the process. Just start again.

12. Group Work or Peer Support

Sometimes it helps to share your struggles with negative thoughts in a group setting or with a trusted peer:

- **Group therapy**: In a safe environment, you can hear how others question their negative thinking, which might inspire you to try new tactics.
- **Peer check-ins**: You and a friend can hold each other accountable. If you text each other daily with one negative thought you faced and how you challenged it, you can cheer each other on.
- **Workshops or classes**: Some community centers offer courses on stress management or CBT basics. These can provide structure to keep practicing.

Hearing others' stories can remind you that negative thoughts are common among people who have faced hard events, but they can be changed over time.

13. Trying New Activities to Shift the Mind

Sometimes, negative thinking is stronger when you feel stuck in the same routines. A fresh activity can open mental space for new perspectives:

1. **Gentle hobbies**: Painting, coloring, or planting small indoor greens can offer a sense of calm and achievement.
2. **Physical movement**: Light exercise, dance, or yoga-style stretches can improve mood and counter thoughts like "I'm too weak" or "I can't do anything."
3. **Learning a skill**: Trying a language app, a craft, or short online classes can show you that you can gain new abilities, pushing back against thoughts of being "useless."
4. **Volunteering**: Helping at a local shelter or community event can shift your focus outward, reminding you that you have something to give.

These activities do not remove your problems, but they break the cycle of negative thoughts and offer moments of healthier self-reflection.

14. Using Humor Carefully

Humor can sometimes lift a negative mood, but it needs to be used carefully:

- **Laughing at small blunders**: If you make a minor mistake, sometimes humor can reduce self-blame. "Well, I spilled my coffee again—maybe I'm testing gravity to be sure it still works!"
- **Watching or reading lighthearted materials**: Gentle comedy shows or funny videos might disrupt a negative thought loop.
- **Avoid harsh self-jokes**: Making fun of yourself in a cruel way can feed negative beliefs. Aim for friendly humor instead.

While humor is not a cure-all, it can create a small break in heavy thinking. If used gently and kindly, it can be part of a larger plan to shift your mood.

---

15. Knowing When to Seek Deeper Help

Sometimes negative thoughts tie closely to deeper wounds that cannot be eased by self-help alone. If you notice:

- **Constant thoughts of self-harm** or that life is not worth living
- **Ongoing paranoia** or the belief that everyone is out to harm you
- **Inability to function** in daily tasks due to anxious or depressive thoughts
- **Thoughts that plague you day and night** with no relief

It may be time to reach out to a counselor or mental health professional. They can guide you through structured methods to ease these patterns. Medications might also be considered if your doctor or psychiatrist believes that could help with severe anxiety or depression.

---

16. Practicing Mindful Observation

Mindfulness is about paying attention to your present experience without judging it. It can help you notice negative thoughts as they arise, then let them pass rather than get stuck:

1. **Observe the thought**: "I just noticed the thought, 'No one likes me.'"
2. **Name any feelings**: "That thought brings up sadness and fear."

3. **Return focus to your breath** or a neutral object in the room.
4. **Let the thought fade**: Picture it like a cloud moving across the sky. You do not chase it or push it away; you just watch it go.

Some people find that regular mindfulness practice reduces the intensity of negative thoughts because the thoughts do not get fed by immediate worry or panic.

---

17. Setting Realistic Goals

Negative thoughts sometimes come from expectations that are too high or from feeling like you are not meeting standards. Setting small, realistic goals can help:

- **Break down tasks**: If you have a big project, split it into steps so you do not think, "I'll never finish."
- **Include rest time**: Build in short breaks to avoid burnout. Burning out often triggers thoughts like "I am too weak."
- **Track progress**: Jot down completed steps, no matter how small. You might see that you actually did more than you thought, which counters negative beliefs of failure.
- **Reward your efforts**: You can acknowledge your progress with small treats or kind words to yourself.

Realistic goals show you can succeed in manageable steps, helping replace negative self-judgments with a more balanced view of what you can accomplish.

---

18. Creating a Plan for Tough Moments

Even with practice, times will come when negative thoughts feel overwhelming—maybe due to a trigger or a stressful event. A plan can guide you:

1. **Warning signs**: Recognize signals that negative thoughts are spiraling—like a tight chest or racing mind.
2. **Immediate tool**: Have one or two go-to coping methods, such as deep breathing or calling a friend.

3. **Safe words**: If you have a partner or close friend, create a word or phrase to let them know you are struggling, so they can step in with calm support.
4. **Short break**: If possible, remove yourself from the stressful environment until you can think more clearly.

A plan helps you react more calmly instead of letting negative thoughts run your actions.

---

19. Tracking Changes in Your Thinking

As weeks and months pass, you may want to check whether your new ways of thinking are paying off:

- **Write down past negative beliefs** you used to have all the time. Are they showing up less now? Are they weaker in intensity?
- **Check emotional changes**: Do you feel a bit less fear, shame, or hopelessness than before? Even a small shift is a sign of progress.
- **Ask close friends**: Sometimes others see improvements before you notice them. They might say, "You seem more confident," or "You don't seem as jumpy."
- **Be kind to yourself**: If you have a setback, it does not erase your gains. Healing rarely goes in a straight line.

Seeing positive changes, no matter how small, can motivate you to keep practicing balanced thinking.

Chapter 14: Helping Others Understand

Healing from trauma often feels like an inside job, but it can be strongly affected by how people around you respond. If they do not understand what PTSD is or why certain events or places are triggering, they might say or do things that unintentionally add to your stress. On the other hand, when friends, family, or coworkers grasp even the basics of what you are going through, they can lend meaningful help. This chapter focuses on how to share your experience with others in a way that encourages understanding, kindness, and practical support. We will talk about picking the right people to open up to, figuring out how much to say, and handling common reactions. We will also explore what to do if someone responds poorly.

---

1. Why Bother Explaining?

It can be tempting to avoid any conversation about trauma. You might fear being judged, doubted, or labeled. However, choosing to help trusted individuals understand can bring benefits:

1. **Reduced isolation**: Secrecy about your trauma can make you feel alone. Sharing with someone safe can provide relief.
2. **Practical help**: If people know your triggers or needs, they can avoid saying certain things or creating stressful environments.
3. **Closer connections**: Letting someone in on your story can deepen your bond, as they see a more honest version of you.
4. **Clearer boundaries**: Explaining your limits—like not wanting to talk about details or needing a calm space—can help others respect those boundaries.

Of course, whether you share is your choice. You do not owe anyone your personal story. The goal is not to give away secrets you do not want to share. Instead, it is to find ways to help people around you interact with you in a more supportive, informed manner.

---

2. Choosing Who to Tell

Not everyone in your life needs to know about your trauma. It is wise to pick certain people who you trust or who influence your daily life. Some factors:

- **Level of closeness**: Are they a close friend, family member, or partner? They might benefit from understanding more because they see you often.
- **Ability to keep confidences**: If the person tends to gossip, maybe they are not the best choice for sharing sensitive details.
- **Emotional maturity**: Some people can listen calmly and respond with empathy. Others may panic, judge, or turn the conversation back to themselves.
- **Relevance**: A coworker or manager might need to know certain boundaries if triggers happen at work. But they do not need all details—only the information that helps them be flexible or respectful.

Start small with one or two individuals who have earned your trust. Over time, you can decide if you feel comfortable expanding that circle.

---

3. Figuring Out What to Say

When opening up about trauma or PTSD, many people worry about giving too much detail or prompting someone to pity them. It helps to plan a bit:

1. **Focus on your needs**: You might say, "I have PTSD, which means I sometimes get really anxious if I hear loud bangs. If you notice me get upset, please give me a moment to do some breathing."
2. **Explain the basics**: A brief mention of what PTSD is can help if they have never heard of it. You might say, "PTSD means my brain stays on alert because of past events. I might have flashbacks or strong fear responses."
3. **Use plain language**: You do not have to teach a psychology lesson. Keep it simple: "Sometimes I have nightmares," or "I get flashbacks of a bad event I lived through."
4. **Avoid graphic details**: Unless you want or need to share them, you can keep descriptions general. For example, "I was in a very scary situation that still affects me. I don't feel ready to talk about the specifics."

The key is to strike a balance: enough information for them to understand your behavior or needs, but not so much that you feel unsafe or overexposed.

---

4. How to Start the Conversation

Picking the right time and place can make these talks smoother:

- **Private setting**: Choose a place where you will not be interrupted, like a quiet room at home or a calm corner of a park.
- **Check their schedule**: Make sure the person you are talking to has time to listen.
- **Ease in**: You might begin with, "There's something important about me I'd like you to know. It's not easy to talk about, but I think it's important that you understand."
- **Watch your comfort level**: If you feel too nervous, you could consider writing a short letter or email, which gives you control over how much you share.

Remember, you have the right to stop or change the subject if it becomes too uncomfortable. You are in control of your story.

---

5. Handling Different Reactions

People can respond in all sorts of ways. Some might be supportive right away, while others may seem unsure what to say. Common reactions include:

1. **Empathy**: They might say, "I'm so sorry you went through that" or "How can I help?"
2. **Shock or discomfort**: They may not know how to reply. This can come across as silence or a quick change of subject.
3. **Questioning**: They might ask, "Why didn't you tell me before?" or "What exactly happened?" They could be curious or worried.
4. **Disbelief or minimization**: Sadly, some people might not believe you, or they might say it "doesn't sound so bad."

If someone reacts poorly, it can be painful. Remind yourself that their response is about them, not about you. A person might lack the emotional tools or knowledge to understand. This does not mean your story or feelings are not valid.

---

6. Educating Them Gently

When a person wants to learn more, you can share additional details:

- **Simple examples**: "Because of my experience, I sometimes jump if someone touches me from behind. It is not that I'm mad at you; it's just my body's reflex."
- **Clarifying triggers**: "Hearing fireworks or popping balloons can remind me of gunshots, which sets off my anxiety."
- **Describing flashbacks**: "A flashback feels like I'm re-living the worst parts of my past. I might look spaced out or very scared. If that happens, you can speak to me calmly or offer me a drink of water."
- **Offering resources**: You could suggest a short article or brochure that explains PTSD basics so they have more background.

Remember, it is not your job to teach them everything about mental health, but sharing a bit of knowledge can reduce confusion and help them be more supportive.

---

7. Involving Them in Your Support System

Once someone understands you face certain challenges, they might ask, "How can I help?" You can offer ideas:

1. **Checking in**: A simple text or call saying, "How are you today?" can mean a lot when you feel isolated.
2. **Respecting boundaries**: If you need quiet time after a panic episode, they can respect that without pushing you to talk.
3. **Helping with daily stress**: Sometimes, practical help like running errands or picking up groceries can ease the load.
4. **Being present**: If you have an anxiety trigger, they can stand by you or guide you to a calmer place.
5. **Listening without judgment**: Remind them that you do not need them to fix your feelings, just to hear you out.

Having a clear role can make your helper feel more confident. They will not guess what you want; they will know exactly how to be supportive.

---

8. Explaining Your Needs at Work or School

If PTSD symptoms affect your job or studies, you might consider telling a supervisor, teacher, or counselor. This can lead to reasonable adjustments:

- **Flexible deadlines** if flashbacks or nightmares disrupt your sleep.
- **Short breaks** during the day to use calming methods.
- **Requesting a quieter workspace** or seat if noise is triggering.
- **Clear communication** so you know about changes in routines or schedules that might add stress.

You are not required to share personal details with a boss or teacher. You can simply say, "I have a condition that affects my stress levels. Could we arrange a short break when I feel overwhelmed?" Many workplaces or schools have policies to assist people with mental health conditions. Knowing your rights can give you confidence in asking for what you need.

---

9. Talking with Children About Your Trauma

If you have children, they might notice you acting differently at times—jumping when a door slams, avoiding certain movies, or crying at night. In such cases:

1. **Use age-appropriate language**: A young child might only need to hear, "Mommy had something scary happen in the past, so she sometimes gets frightened."
2. **Reassure them**: Make sure they know they are safe, and you are getting help to feel better.
3. **Invite questions**: Kids might ask, "What happened?" or "Will it happen to me?" You can give simple, honest answers without going into detail that might upset them.
4. **Teach them signals**: Let them know if you have a sign or word that means you need a moment to calm down. Encourage them not to feel guilty if they see you upset.

Being open at their level can reduce confusion and help them see that scary feelings can be talked about and managed.

---

10. Cultural and Community Factors

Some cultures do not openly discuss mental health or trauma. You might face extra hurdles:

- **Fear of stigma**: Relatives or community members might judge PTSD as a weakness or shameful.
- **Language barriers**: Explaining PTSD symptoms could be harder if there is no similar term in your language.
- **Seeking alternative help**: Some communities rely on spiritual or community-led solutions rather than therapy.

If you sense stigma, you could try sharing just enough information to get practical support without revealing every detail. Also, look for groups or counselors who understand your culture, as they might offer more sensitive ways to talk about your experiences.

---

11. Dealing with Disbelief or Hurtful Comments

Not everyone will respond with kindness. Some might say, "That was so long ago—get over it," or "You're exaggerating." Here are ways to handle negative responses:

1. **Set boundaries**: Calmly state, "I understand you don't see it the same way, but this is real for me, and I won't continue this discussion if you dismiss my feelings."
2. **End the conversation**: If someone refuses to show respect, you can walk away or change the subject.
3. **Find your support elsewhere**: Put your energy into relationships where you feel safe and understood.
4. **Remind yourself**: Their disbelief does not change the truth of what you went through. They might be uncomfortable or lack empathy.

It is painful when someone reacts with judgment or mockery. Seek comfort with a friend or counselor, reinforcing that their response is a reflection of them, not you.

---

12. Building Communication Skills

Sharing about trauma can be intense. Practicing clear communication can help:

- **Use "I" statements**: "I feel anxious when I hear sudden loud noises" instead of "You always scare me." This keeps blame out of the conversation.
- **Stay calm if possible**: Speaking slowly, keeping your tone steady—these can help the other person remain calm too.
- **Ask for feedback**: "Do you understand what I mean by flashbacks? Does it make sense when I say I need a quick break sometimes?"
- **Explain your goals**: "I don't want pity; I just want you to know why I might leave a room suddenly."

Respectful, clear language improves the chance that people will truly hear what you are saying.

---

13. Knowing Your Limits

Even if someone is kind, rehashing your trauma can be draining. It is okay to set limits:

- **Shorten the conversation**: If you start feeling overwhelmed, you can say, "I need to pause here, but I appreciate you listening."
- **Focus on the present**: You do not have to detail the past event. It might be enough to say, "Because of what happened before, these are the symptoms I deal with now."
- **Decline certain topics**: If someone pushes for details, you can respond, "I'm not comfortable discussing that part."
- **Give partial information**: You can reveal that you experienced a serious accident or betrayal without describing exactly how it happened.

Setting these boundaries protects you from being retraumatized by constant retelling of the story.

---

14. Explaining Triggers and Safety Plans

If you trust someone, it might help to be more specific about triggers or what to do if you have a flashback:

1. **Name the triggers**: "I get triggered by shouting. If voices get loud, I might panic or leave the room."
2. **Outline your coping methods**: "When I am triggered, I try deep breathing or stepping outside. If you see me doing that, please give me space until I say I am okay to talk."
3. **Request specific help**: "If I seem stuck in a flashback, it helps if you call my name calmly and remind me where I am."
4. **Explain what not to do**: "Please don't grab me suddenly, and don't tell me to 'snap out of it.' That might scare me more."

Giving people a roadmap can reduce confusion and help them respond in a supportive way.

---

15. Sharing Accomplishments and Progress

When talking to others, do not only focus on the hard parts of trauma. You can also mention improvements or coping successes. Let's avoid words we were told not to use, but we can say:

- **"I managed my anxiety well last week by going for short walks."**
- **"I am proud of how I spoke up for myself when I felt uneasy."**
- **"I tried a new relaxation video, and it seemed to help me sleep better."**

By including these positive notes, you show people that, yes, trauma is part of your life, but you are actively working on growth. It can also invite them to cheer you on.

---

16. Role of Professional Mediators or Family Therapy

In some cases, the misunderstanding is so deep that sitting everyone down with a professional mediator or family therapist can help:

- **Neutral environment**: A therapist's office can be a safer place to discuss painful topics with structured guidance.
- **Clarifying misunderstandings**: A counselor can help family members see that your triggers or avoidance are not personal attacks but rooted in PTSD.
- **Learning communication tools**: The therapist might suggest ways for you and your loved ones to handle future conflicts or tense moments.

This approach can be especially helpful if family conflict is fueling your stress or if certain relatives downplay your trauma.

17. Helping Others Understand They Are Not to Blame

Sometimes parents, partners, or close friends feel guilty, thinking they should have protected you or done something differently. If it helps you, you can gently reassure them:

- **"It happened because of the situation, not because you failed."**
- **"You did not know what was going on at the time."**
- **"I appreciate that you care. Right now, the best way to help is by understanding my needs."**

Making sure they do not carry misguided blame can prevent further emotional strain on your relationships.

18. Technology and Social Media

Some people share parts of their trauma story on social media, hoping for support. This can connect you with understanding folks, but consider:

- **Privacy risks**: Once posted, personal details can spread beyond your control.
- **Unexpected responses**: Public forums might bring negativity or doubt.
- **Check group rules**: If you join a support group online, be sure it is well-moderated and respectful.
- **Direct messages**: You might prefer private chats with trusted individuals over broad public posts.

If you do share online, think carefully about how much detail you want to reveal and whether the platform is safe from trolling or harassment.

---

19. Steady Understanding Over Time

People may not "get it" instantly. They might need gentle reminders about what triggers are or why you sometimes cancel plans at the last minute. Be patient but also firm in your boundaries:

- **Repeat key points** if they forget. For instance, "Remember that large crowds make me uneasy, so I might leave early."
- **Show gratitude** when someone respects your needs. A simple thank-you can reinforce positive behavior.
- **Keep lines open**: If they have questions, invite them to ask in a calm, respectful way.
- **Know your limit**: If someone repeatedly ignores your explanations, consider whether this person can be part of your close circle.

Over time, consistent communication can create a more caring environment where you feel safer.

Chapter 15: Overcoming Avoidance

Avoidance can be a strong force for people dealing with Post-Traumatic Stress Disorder (PTSD) or trauma-related stress. You might notice you steer clear of anything that reminds you of your painful experience—places, conversations, smells, or activities. Sometimes avoidance feels like the only way to stay safe. But it can also shrink your life, making you miss important events or lose out on things you used to enjoy. This chapter will look at what avoidance is, why it happens, and how you can face the things you have been dodging in a way that feels safe and steady. By learning to handle avoidance, you can rebuild control over your daily life without constantly running from triggers.

1. Understanding Avoidance

Avoidance can show up in many ways:

- **Physical avoidance**: Not going to a certain neighborhood, store, or even skipping doctor appointments if they bring up bad memories.
- **Emotional avoidance**: Refusing to talk or think about the event, shutting down emotions that feel scary or sad.
- **Situational avoidance**: Steering clear of news stories, social gatherings, or other everyday moments that might hold triggers.

In some cases, this avoidance can become so big that it seems like life revolves around staying away from anything that might spark fear or sadness. While this might seem to lower stress in the moment, it can also keep you stuck, unable to heal from what happened because you never get a chance to see that you can handle your feelings or triggers.

2. Why Avoidance Happens

After trauma, your mind and body want to protect you from feeling that same hurt again. Avoidance is part of that protective instinct:

1. **Fear of flashbacks**: If remembering the event feels overwhelming, you might avoid anything that brings it to mind.

2. **Fear of strong emotions**: Sadness, anger, or shame can be so intense that you would rather not go near them at all.
3. **Feeling "safer" alone**: Sometimes, being around people or places might remind you of past harm. Staying away might feel like the safest option.
4. **Worry about losing control**: You might think, "If I face this, I will have a breakdown," so you sidestep it instead.

Though avoidance can offer short-term relief, it usually extends the trauma's reach, because it keeps you living in fear of what might trigger you.

---

3. Signs That Avoidance Is Getting in the Way

It can be hard to notice how big avoidance has become in your life. Some clues:

- **You plan your day around avoiding certain places or people**.
- **You stop doing hobbies** that you once loved because they might stir up old memories.
- **You have trouble talking about the past at all**, even in therapy or with someone you trust.
- **You often feel numb** or disconnected from others, as if your emotions are locked away.
- **Your world seems to be shrinking**, with fewer activities and social connections.

When avoidance reaches this level, it does more harm than good. It keeps you from trying new things or healing from old wounds.

---

4. The Cycle of Avoidance and Anxiety

Avoidance might feel like it lowers anxiety in the moment, but it often strengthens fear in the long run:

1. **Encounter a Trigger**: You sense or see something that reminds you of the trauma.
2. **Anxiety Rises**: Your heart races, your muscles tense, or your mind fills with worry.
3. **Avoid It**: You leave the situation or push the thoughts away.

4. **Short-Term Relief**: You feel calmer because the trigger is gone—for now.
5. **Reinforced Fear**: The next time the trigger shows up, your anxiety might spike even higher, convincing you that avoidance is "necessary."

This cycle can become very strong. The key to breaking it is learning safe, steady ways to face the triggers or feelings until they lose some of their power.

---

5. Slowly Facing Avoided Situations: Exposure

"Exposure" is a term often used in therapy for gently and gradually facing the things you want to avoid. This does not mean jumping straight into the hardest scenario. Instead, you move in small steps:

1. **List what you avoid**: Write down places, activities, or topics that spark anxiety.
2. **Rank them by difficulty**: Give each avoided thing a score from 1 (slightly uncomfortable) to 10 (extremely upsetting).
3. **Start with low or middle items**: Pick something that is challenging but not overwhelmingly so.
4. **Plan a small step**: If you have been avoiding grocery stores, maybe first look at pictures of a store. Next time, drive near the store but do not go in. Then walk inside briefly, and leave if anxiety gets too high.
5. **Use coping skills**: Practice breathing or grounding exercises before, during, and after each step.
6. **Repeat**: As you do the same step multiple times, you often realize the fear intensity decreases. Then you can move to a slightly harder step.

Exposure can be done with help from a therapist or on your own if you feel prepared. The purpose is to see that while triggers are uncomfortable, they are not always as dangerous as your mind expects.

---

6. Handling Emotional Avoidance

It is not just places or situations we avoid—many of us also dodge emotions like sadness, anger, or guilt. Emotional avoidance might look like:

- **Shutting down** or "numbing out" when certain feelings arise.

- **Using distractions** like constant TV, social media, or working too many hours to avoid being alone with your thoughts.
- **Refusing to talk about topics** that might make you cry or get angry.

Yet refusing to feel emotions can lead to a bottled-up state where you experience numbness or sudden outbursts. To face emotional avoidance:

1. **Name the feeling**: Label it: "I am feeling sadness right now," or "This is anger."
2. **Allow a small window**: Let yourself sit with that emotion for a minute or two. Notice the physical sensations, like tightness in your chest.
3. **Practice safe release**: You might write about the emotion, talk with a friend, or allow yourself a brief cry.
4. **Stop if overwhelmed**: If it becomes too intense, shift to a coping skill (breathing, distraction) and try again later.

Learning to feel without being swallowed up by emotions is a skill, and it grows with practice.

---

7. Coping Tools for Facing What You Avoid

Before trying to expose yourself to a feared situation, it helps to have a set of coping skills ready:

- **Grounding exercises**: Use your senses to stay in the present (such as the 5-4-3-2-1 method).
- **Deep breathing**: Inhale slowly and count to four, hold for four, exhale for four, then rest briefly.
- **Positive self-talk**: Remind yourself, "I can leave if I need to," or "I've handled hard things before."
- **Buddy system**: Take a trusted friend along or have them on standby by phone.
- **Relaxation music**: Listening to calm music before or after facing a trigger can reduce tension.

Having these tools in place gives you the confidence to step into what you have been avoiding because you know you have ways to handle panic if it arises.

---

8. Creating a Step-by-Step Exposure Plan

Let's imagine a common avoidance scenario: someone is scared of going to a mall because it reminds them of a past traumatic event. A step-by-step plan might look like:

1. **Look at photos of the mall** on your phone or computer. Rate your anxiety. Practice breathing until it lowers.
2. **Drive by the mall parking lot** but do not go inside. Stay a few minutes, use grounding if anxious, then leave.
3. **Walk around the outside of the mall** briefly. If panic rises, practice your coping skills.
4. **Enter the mall for a short time**—maybe go to just one store or a café.
5. **Add time inside**: Each visit can be a bit longer, or involve more areas.
6. **Evaluate progress**: If one step feels okay, move to the next. If it remains too distressing, repeat it until anxiety lessens.

Going slowly helps you see that your body can handle the discomfort and that nothing truly harmful is happening now.

---

9. Balancing Courage and Caution

Facing avoidance does not mean forcing yourself to do something too big before you are ready. It is about a balance:

- **Pushing gently**: Growth often requires stepping outside your comfort zone, even if it feels scary.
- **Not overwhelming yourself**: Jumping into a 10-level fear when you have not managed a 4 or 5 yet might lead to panic and reinforce avoidance.
- **Using rest days**: After an intense exposure practice, it might help to take a day or two to focus on calming or enjoyable activities.

A steady pace can lead to real change without pushing you into a meltdown.

---

10. Dealing with Setbacks in Exposure

Sometimes you might feel ready to face a trigger, but panic creeps back in. You may leave sooner than planned or decide not to try that day. This is okay:

- **Remember it is not failure**: Avoidance patterns are deep. Breaking them can lead to two steps forward, one step back.
- **Reflect calmly**: Ask yourself, "Which part was too overwhelming? Did I move too fast or forget to use my coping tools?"
- **Try again** with an adjusted plan. Maybe you aim for a shorter time or bring a friend for support.
- **Be kind to yourself**: Remind yourself that this process can take time.

Setbacks are normal in healing. They do not mean you are stuck forever, only that you might need to adjust your methods.

---

11. Partnering with a Therapist for Exposure Work

If avoidance is severe, or you do not feel comfortable doing exposure on your own, working with a therapist can help:

- **Safety and guidance**: A trained counselor understands how to gradually introduce triggers without pushing you too far.
- **Structured approach**: They might use specific methods like Prolonged Exposure Therapy, where you talk through or imagine the traumatic event in small, guided sessions.
- **Accountability**: Having someone to check in with can keep you motivated and steady.
- **Practice coping skills**: Therapists can teach and help you rehearse your skills, so you feel confident using them outside of sessions.

Knowing you have professional backup can make all the difference when facing scary memories or situations.

---

12. Handling Avoidance in Relationships

Sometimes, avoidance can lead you to keep a distance from friends, family, or partners because you worry about being judged or overwhelmed. Overcoming this might involve:

1. **Sharing your feelings**: Explain, "I've been pulling away because I'm scared of feeling too vulnerable."

2. **Setting clear boundaries**: You can let loved ones know which topics are off-limits for now, or how much time you need alone.
3. **Practicing small doses**: Maybe you join a short get-together instead of avoiding social events altogether.
4. **Asking for understanding**: If someone knows you are dealing with triggers, they might be more supportive when you need breaks or suddenly leave a room.

Reconnecting with people can help you feel less isolated, which is vital for long-term healing.

---

13. Overcoming Avoidance of Medical or Professional Care

It is common for trauma survivors to avoid doctors, dentists, or other professionals, especially if past experiences were frightening. To face this:

- **Choose a caring provider**: Seek out someone known for gentle bedside manners or who has worked with trauma survivors.
- **Bring a support person**: A friend or relative in the waiting room can lower anxiety.
- **Communicate needs**: Tell the doctor or nurse, "I feel anxious; please explain each step before you do it."
- **Schedule shorter visits**: If possible, have multiple shorter appointments instead of one long session.
- **Use coping tools**: Practice grounding or deep breathing in the office if anxiety rises.

Addressing health issues is crucial. Avoidance can lead to untreated problems, making life harder down the road.

---

14. Facing Trauma-Related Tasks

Certain tasks may directly remind you of trauma—like filling out paperwork that asks about past experiences, or driving by the site of an accident. Strategies include:

1. **Break down the task**: Complete one part of the form at a time, or drive a small portion of the route each day.
2. **Reward yourself**: After facing part of the task, do something calming or pleasant.
3. **Enlist help**: A friend can sit with you while you fill out forms or offer to drive you partway.
4. **Plan extra downtime**: Emotional tasks can be draining. Make sure to rest or do self-care afterward.

Step by step, you show yourself that you can handle these tasks without being trapped by panic.

---

15. Recognizing Healthy Avoidance vs. Harmful Avoidance

Sometimes you truly do need to avoid things for your well-being. For example, avoiding an unsafe person who hurt you is wise, not harmful. So how do you tell the difference?

- **Healthy avoidance**: Protecting yourself from real threats or unhealthy situations (like staying away from someone who is abusive).
- **Harmful avoidance**: Fleeing from safe situations that remind you of trauma or feelings, but which pose no real danger now.

Check if the thing you are avoiding is actually a genuine threat. If it is not, maybe it is time to reconsider. Avoiding all potential reminders can keep you locked in fear.

---

16. What If You Never Feel "Ready"?

You might be waiting to feel completely brave before facing what you avoid. However, you may never feel perfectly ready. Change often requires taking a leap of faith:

- **Recognize readiness is rarely 100%**: Even a small part of you that thinks, "I can try," might be enough.
- **Use partial steps**: If you can only manage half of your plan, that is still progress.

- **Expect mixed feelings**: It is normal to feel fear and courage at the same time.
- **Be proud of attempts**: Trying at all is already a break from total avoidance.

Moving forward despite lingering nerves is a big part of growth. You do not have to be fearless, only willing to see what happens if you face what you have been avoiding.

---

17. Self-Talk During Tough Moments

When stepping into something you have avoided, your inner voice can either help or hinder:

- **Helpful thoughts**: "I can handle my anxiety," "I can leave anytime," "This feeling will pass."
- **Harmful thoughts**: "I'm trapped," "I'm going to lose control," "I shouldn't have tried."

Pay attention to your mental chatter. If it gets negative, gently replace it with calmer, reassuring statements. You do not have to believe them 100% at first. Over time, they become more convincing.

---

18. Learning from Each Experience

After each attempt to face avoidance, reflect on what you learned:

- **What helped?** Maybe focusing on your breath or having a friend nearby really worked.
- **What was hard?** Notice if a specific sound or thought triggered a spike in fear.
- **How intense was your anxiety before and after?** Even if it was high at the start, maybe it dropped by the end.
- **Do you feel a bit more confident now?** Recognizing gains helps you build a sense of mastery.

No matter how big or small the exposure was, each experience can guide your next steps.

Chapter 16: Everyday Strategies for Healing

When living with trauma or Post-Traumatic Stress Disorder (PTSD), progress does not only happen in therapy sessions or during big breakthroughs. Much of it happens in the small, daily choices you make—from how you start your morning to what you do before you go to sleep. Everyday strategies can help create a sense of calm and stability, even when life feels unsettled. This chapter looks at practical ways to handle day-to-day stress, stay connected to your well-being, and build a lifestyle that supports your mind and body. These strategies are not fancy or complicated, yet they can make a real difference over time.

1. Why Everyday Routines Matter

Routines can bring comfort and predictability, especially when trauma leaves you feeling that everything is unsafe or out of control. Small routines or habits can:

1. **Reduce decision fatigue**: Having regular times to eat, rest, or do chores means you do not have to think about them too much.
2. **Build a sense of achievement**: Each time you keep a simple routine, like brushing your teeth at the same hour, you show yourself you can follow through on tasks.
3. **Lower anxiety**: Predictable habits can reassure your mind that not every moment is a crisis, which can help calm the body's constant alertness.
4. **Create structure**: Even if your life feels chaotic, routines act like anchors, keeping you from drifting too far into stress.

A routine does not have to be rigid. It is about gentle predictability, not forcing yourself to follow a strict schedule. You can adapt routines to your energy level and the realities of your day.

2. Starting the Morning with Calm

Mornings can set the tone for the entire day. When you have PTSD, you might wake up feeling anxious or weighed down by bad dreams. A calming morning plan can help you begin on steadier ground. Some ideas include:

- **Wake up at a regular time**: If possible, avoid constantly changing your wake-up hour. Consistency helps your body's internal clock.
- **Stretch or do light movement**: A few minutes of gentle stretching, slow walking around your home, or easy body movements can loosen tense muscles and get blood flowing.
- **Simple breathing practice**: Before picking up your phone or leaving your bed, try a short breathing exercise. Inhale deeply for four counts, hold for four, exhale for four, then rest briefly. Doing this a few times can clear lingering night worries.
- **Pick a mindful activity**: This might be brewing tea, noticing its smell and warmth, or reading a brief, calming passage.

None of these steps need to be long. Even a couple of minutes can help you ground yourself, signaling your mind that you are stepping into the day gently instead of jumping straight into stress.

---

3. Balancing Daily Tasks and Rest

After trauma, daily tasks can feel overwhelming. You might struggle with chores or errands that once seemed simple. Here are ways to keep up without burning out:

1. **Use to-do lists wisely**: Write down only a few key tasks rather than pages of them. Seeing a huge list can cause more stress.
2. **Divide larger tasks**: If laundry or cleaning feels like too much, focus on just one part—wash a single load or clean one corner of the kitchen.
3. **Schedule short breaks**: Take five-minute pauses every hour or two. Stretch, sip water, or step outside briefly if you can. Small breaks can reset your mind and lower tension.
4. **Avoid perfection**: Aim for "good enough." Pressuring yourself to get everything perfect can worsen anxiety.
5. **Alternate stressful tasks with easier ones**: After doing something demanding—like paying bills—do a simpler task, like tidying a small drawer or taking out the trash.

This approach builds a balance between doing what needs to be done and allowing your body and mind the rest they need.

---

4. Healthy Eating Habits

Trauma can affect appetite in two ways: it might make you lose interest in food or drive you to overeat for comfort. Some ideas to stay nourished:

- **Plan basic meals**: You do not need to cook gourmet dishes. Simple, balanced meals—like chicken (or beans) with vegetables and rice—can be enough.
- **Keep easy snacks available**: Fruits, nuts, yogurt cups, or similar items can give you a quick boost when you have no energy to cook.
- **Watch caffeine and sugar**: They can worsen anxiety if taken in large amounts. Try to keep them moderate and notice how they affect your mood.
- **Try mindful eating**: When possible, avoid screens during meals. Pay attention to the taste and texture of your food. This can help prevent overeating or forgetting that you have already eaten.
- **Stay hydrated**: Dehydration can cause headaches and irritability, which add to stress.

Food does not have to be perfect. The main goal is to keep a steady intake of nutrients, so your body has the fuel it needs to cope with daily challenges.

---

5. Scheduling Movement Throughout the Day

Physical movement can help lower stress hormones and improve mood. But you do not have to do intense workouts. Many trauma survivors find gentler options more manageable:

1. **Short walks**: Going outside (if it is safe) for even 10 minutes can help clear your head. If you cannot go outdoors, pacing indoors works, too.
2. **Stretch breaks**: Standing up to stretch your arms, shoulders, and back every hour or two can reduce tension.
3. **Simple home exercises**: Try easy chair exercises or follow a brief, beginner-friendly online video.
4. **Focus on comfort**: If a gym setting is too overwhelming, movement at home or in a quiet outdoor space might feel better.

Getting some movement each day can release built-up energy and help with sleep. Remember to respect your body's limits and any physical conditions.

6. Relaxation and Quiet Time

When dealing with PTSD, your mind might stay on high alert. Scheduling moments of rest can help calm the system:

- **Set a relaxation reminder**: Put an alarm on your phone a couple of times a day to pause for calming exercises, such as slow breathing or listening to soft music.
- **Explore gentle relaxation methods**: These could be guided meditations, progressive muscle relaxation, or nature sounds.
- **Create a "quiet corner"**: A spot in your home with cushions or a chair where you can sit, read, or listen to calming sounds without disturbance.
- **Limit constant noise**: If background noise makes you anxious, try using noise-cancelling headphones or playing soothing background music at a gentle volume.

Quiet time is not a luxury; it is a way to tell your nervous system that it is safe to turn down the internal alarm.

7. Using Grounding Activities

Grounding activities pull your focus to the present moment, steering you away from distressing memories or fears of the future. Some easy grounding methods:

1. **5-4-3-2-1 Method**: Name five things you can see, four you can touch, three you can hear, two you can smell, and one you can taste (or imagine tasting).
2. **Hold an object**: Pick up something small—a smooth stone, a stress ball, or a piece of fabric—and notice its texture, temperature, and shape.
3. **Listen intently**: Stop and identify the sounds around you—like humming appliances, distant traffic, or birds.
4. **Focus on your feet**: Notice how your feet feel against the floor, the weight in your heels, or any pressure points.

These exercises can be done anytime you feel anxious or disconnected, reminding you that you are in the here and now, not in the traumatic past.

8. Staying Connected with Others

Isolation is common with trauma, but friendly contact can ease stress and loneliness:

- **Check in with someone daily**: Send a short message or make a quick call. It does not have to be a long chat, just a sign of connection.
- **Plan low-key meetups**: If big gatherings are too much, invite a friend for coffee or a walk. Keep it short if needed.
- **Join supportive groups**: Local or online groups for people dealing with PTSD or stress can help you feel less alone.
- **Set boundaries**: If you need alone time, say so kindly. Let people know you value their presence but also need space.

Staying connected can remind you that you are not facing everything by yourself. Even small interactions can lift your spirits.

---

9. Adding Creative or Enjoyable Outlets

Trauma often steals joy from daily life. Reintroducing fun or creative tasks, even if small, can brighten your mood:

1. **Try simple art**: Doodling, coloring, or painting with basic tools. Focus on the colors and shapes rather than producing perfect art.
2. **Listen to music**: Pick tunes that soothe you. Some prefer soft piano music; others might like nature sounds or gentle guitar.
3. **Light crafting**: Activities like knitting, clay modeling, or making bracelets can keep hands busy and help calm the mind.
4. **Explore safe hobbies**: If certain hobbies used to bring you joy, consider whether you can try them in a modified or shorter form now.

These outlets are not meant to distract you from healing but to remind you that life can hold pleasant moments alongside the hard ones.

---

10. Keeping a Journal or Tracker

Writing down your experiences can help you notice progress or patterns:

- **Daily mood check**: Rate your mood or stress on a simple scale from 1 (calm) to 10 (very stressed).
- **List triggers**: If something upset you, note what happened, how you felt, and any coping methods you tried.
- **Track positives**: Maybe you found a new coping skill that helped or you got out of bed sooner than usual. Write these little wins down.
- **Use bullet points**: You do not need long paragraphs. A few words each day can be enough to see trends over time.

Journaling helps you see that you are not stagnant. Even on tough days, there might be small victories you can recognize in writing.

11. Setting Realistic Goals for Each Day

When dealing with PTSD, even small goals can feel big:

1. **Choose one or two main tasks**: Examples might be cooking a meal or tidying a part of your living area.
2. **Allow for flexibility**: If you wake up feeling very anxious, reduce the goal or break it into smaller pieces.
3. **Give yourself credit**: Remind yourself that even small tasks count when you are dealing with trauma.
4. **Adjust goals over time**: As you feel more stable, you can try slightly bigger tasks.

Keeping your goals small and doable can lower the risk of feeling overwhelmed. Over time, these little tasks add up.

12. Building Short Breaks into Work or School

If you have a job or you are studying, stress can build up quickly. You might feel triggered by noise, deadlines, or unexpected events. Some strategies:

- **Brief breathing pauses**: Every couple of hours, close your eyes (if it is safe) and take three slow breaths.
- **Stretch at your desk**: Roll your shoulders, stretch your arms, or gently twist your torso. These small movements can release tension.

- **Step outside if possible**: A short walk or even standing in a corridor for a minute can refresh your mind.
- **Use earplugs or headphones**: If loud sounds unsettle you, consider soft earplugs or music at a volume that does not distract you from your tasks.

Regular micro-breaks help you reset rather than letting stress accumulate until it feels unmanageable.

---

13. Safe Evening and Bedtime Routines

Nighttime can be tough for people with PTSD, often due to nightmares or racing thoughts. A calming bedtime routine might include:

1. **Lower lighting**: Dim lights can signal your body to wind down.
2. **Avoid stimulating media**: Scary or action-packed shows close to bedtime might raise anxiety. Switch to gentler content or read something light.
3. **Gentle stretches or relaxation**: A few simple stretches or a short guided relaxation audio can help release built-up tension.
4. **Write down worries**: If thoughts about tomorrow's tasks or past events swirl, jot them on paper. This can ease mental clutter.
5. **Aim for consistent sleep times**: Go to bed at roughly the same hour and wake at a similar time if you can. This steadiness supports better rest.

Even if nightmares still occur, these habits can lower overall nighttime stress and help you fall asleep more peacefully.

---

14. Mindful Technology Use

Smartphones and the internet can be helpful but also overwhelming. Consider:

- **Time limits on news and social media**: Constantly reading distressing headlines or negative comments can spike your anxiety.
- **Set device-free zones**: Choose parts of the day—such as early morning or late evening—when you step away from your phone.
- **Use apps that assist well-being**: Some apps guide relaxation, sleep sounds, or simple meditations.
- **Mute notifications**: Constant pings and buzzes can keep your body on alert. Turning off non-essential notifications can reduce stress.

Mindful use of technology means staying aware of how it affects your feelings and adjusting as needed.

---

15. Checking In with Yourself

It is easy to get lost in tasks and triggers. Creating short check-ins can keep you aware of how you feel:

1. **Morning check-in**: Ask, "How am I feeling physically? Mentally?" If you notice extra tension, maybe do some quick stretches.
2. **Midday check-in**: Pause and see if you need a snack, water, or a moment of quiet.
3. **Evening check-in**: Reflect on the day. Did you handle stress well? Do you need to release any pent-up feelings before bed, maybe by writing them down?

These brief check-ins prevent you from ignoring signs of anxiety or exhaustion until they grow too large.

---

16. Being Kind to Yourself

Self-compassion is an everyday strategy, not just an idea:

- **Use gentle words**: If you catch yourself thinking, "I should be over this," try to switch to, "I'm doing the best I can right now."
- **Allow mistakes**: If a coping strategy does not work one day, you can try again tomorrow.
- **Avoid harsh comparisons**: Comparing your progress to someone else's can fuel discouragement. Each person's trauma and healing are unique.
- **Acknowledge your efforts**: Even if you only managed half of what you wanted, you still took steps. That counts.

Being kind to yourself helps reduce the extra stress that comes from negative self-talk, letting your energy go toward real healing work.

---

17. Preparing for Unexpected Stress

Life does not always follow plans, and triggers can pop up when you least expect. Try these tactics:

1. **Have a go-to grounding method**: If your anxiety spikes, you can do a quick body scan or 5-4-3-2-1 method.
2. **Carry calming tools**: Keep a smooth stone, a small scented lotion, or a stress ball in your bag or pocket.
3. **Develop a signal with a friend**: If you are out together, agree on a word or sign that tells them you are overwhelmed. They can help you find a calmer spot.
4. **Remind yourself you can leave**: If a situation becomes too stressful, it is okay to step out or take a quick break to regroup.

Being ready for surprises does not mean you will never feel anxiety. But it can lower the impact when something catches you off guard.

---

18. Building on Good Days, Handling Bad Days

With PTSD, some days might feel almost normal, while others might be filled with triggers. Everyday strategies can adapt to both:

- **On better days**: Take note of what helps you feel more stable. Maybe you got enough rest or did a fun activity. Keep building those habits.
- **On harder days**: Let yourself scale back. Do not blame yourself if you need more rest or skip non-essential tasks. Return to your core coping methods.
- **Maintain consistency**: Even if you feel good, continue your calming routines. This steadiness can cushion you when a rough day appears.

Good and bad days are both part of the process, but everyday strategies can keep you from falling too hard when stress climbs.

Chapter 17: Handling Setbacks

Living with trauma or PTSD is not a simple climb from low points to brighter days. Instead, it can feel like a winding road with ups and downs. You might have weeks where you manage triggers well, and then—suddenly—an incident or flashback sends you reeling. These hard moments, sometimes called "setbacks," can make you think all your progress is lost. But setbacks are not a sign of failure; they are a normal part of the healing process. This chapter focuses on why setbacks happen, how to address them without adding shame or panic, and how they can even help you grow stronger in the long run.

---

1. Understanding the Nature of Setbacks

A setback occurs when anxiety, nightmares, flashbacks, or avoidance issues flare up again after a period of calm or improvement. Sometimes a clear trigger, like an anniversary of the traumatic event, starts it. Other times it happens without warning. Common feelings during a setback include:

- **Frustration**: "I thought I was doing better. Why am I back here?"
- **Shame**: "I must be weak or failing."
- **Hopelessness**: "Maybe healing is not possible for me."
- **Anger**: "It is unfair that this came back to haunt me."

But in reality, a setback is just a spike in symptoms, not a permanent return to square one. You still have the coping skills and understanding you gained earlier. It is just harder to access them when emotions run high.

---

2. Common Causes of Setbacks

Setbacks can have many triggers:

1. **Anniversaries or dates**: The time of year or month the trauma happened might stir memories.
2. **Stressful life changes**: Things like moving, changing jobs, or dealing with illness can wear down your emotional reserves.

3. **Unexpected reminders**: A sudden loud noise, a TV show with content similar to your trauma, or running into someone who hurt you can trigger intense feelings.
4. **Overwork or burnout**: If you have been pushing yourself too hard and not resting, your coping ability may drop.
5. **Physical health dips**: Lack of sleep, poor nutrition, or illness can weaken resilience.

Seeing these causes is helpful because it reminds you that setbacks often happen for a reason, not because you did something wrong.

---

3. Recognizing Warning Signs Early

Sometimes, there are clues that a setback is coming:

- **Increased irritability**: You might find small annoyances set you off more than usual.
- **Rising anxiety**: A general sense of dread or more frequent panic symptoms.
- **Trouble sleeping again**: Nightmares or insomnia might return or worsen.
- **Feeling numb**: Emotional numbness can show that you are disconnecting to avoid pain.
- **Avoiding daily tasks**: You might skip appointments or ignore chores if you sense triggers.

Catching these signals allows you to act early, using coping skills before things get too overwhelming.

---

4. Responding to a Setback in the Moment

When you notice that a setback has arrived, it is normal to feel discouraged. But rather than panic, try to:

1. **Pause and breathe**: Give yourself a moment to calm the initial surge of fear or shame.
2. **Acknowledge what is happening**: "I am in a setback. My symptoms are up right now."

3. **Use grounding or calming methods**: Try deep breathing, the 5-4-3-2-1 technique, or muscle relaxation to reduce immediate distress.
4. **Speak kindly to yourself**: Remind yourself, "I have been through rough times before, and I can use what I learned."
5. **Consider environment**: If you are in a triggering place, see if you can move somewhere quieter or safer.

The first step is often just gaining enough calm to think clearly about your next move.

---

5. Avoiding Self-Blame

One of the hardest parts of a setback is the self-blame. You might hear an inner voice saying, "I messed up," or "I'm weak." But setbacks do not mean you failed. A more supportive way to look at it is:

- **Trauma healing is uneven**: Symptoms ebb and flow, and that is expected.
- **You have not lost your skills**: They might feel buried under stress, but they are still there.
- **Shame makes things worse**: Blaming yourself can intensify anxiety or depression.
- **Focus on problem-solving**: Instead of criticizing yourself, consider how to soothe symptoms and what might have triggered them.

It helps to see a setback as part of the process, not a reflection of your worth or ability.

---

6. Short-Term Coping During a Setback

When a setback arrives, immediate coping might look like:

1. **Refresher on coping tools**: Revisit your list of grounding methods, calming apps, or supportive contacts.
2. **Daily checklists**: If you are struggling to keep up with chores or responsibilities, make a small, realistic list each morning.
3. **Safe distractions**: Watching a lighthearted show, coloring, or doing a puzzle can give your mind a rest if anxiety spikes.

4. **Social support**: Reach out to a friend, family member, or helpline. It is okay to say, "I am having a rough time right now. Can we talk or text?"
5. **Physical relaxation**: Warm baths, gentle stretches, or a brief walk can help reduce tension in your muscles and mind.

These short-term actions do not fix everything, but they provide a buffer while you ride out the surge in symptoms.

---

7. Reassessing Your Daily Habits

A setback might be a sign that certain daily habits need adjustment:

- **Are you getting enough sleep?** Poor rest can weaken resilience.
- **Have you been skipping meals or eating poorly?** This can spike anxiety.
- **Is your schedule overloaded?** Too many demands might push your stress too high.
- **Are you isolating from everyone?** Avoidance can worsen negative thoughts.

Reflect on your routines. You might need to slow down, cut back on extra tasks, or reconnect with supportive people.

---

8. Using Therapy or Professional Help

If the setback feels intense or lasts longer than expected, consider reconnecting with professional help:

1. **Schedule a tune-up session**: Even if you had finished therapy, a few sessions for support can help.
2. **Try a new approach**: If you have never tried certain methods like EMDR or group therapy, maybe a setback is a sign to explore them.
3. **Medication check**: If you are on medication, talk to your prescribing doctor. Adjustments might be needed if symptoms are flaring.
4. **Crisis resources**: If you feel unsafe or have thoughts of self-harm, call a crisis line or seek immediate help. You are not alone.

Professional guidance can remind you of tools you might have forgotten and offer fresh strategies.

9. Learning from Triggers

A setback might reveal new triggers you did not realize were part of your trauma response. Rather than avoid them forever, you can:

1. **Name the trigger**: "I realized that large social gatherings trigger me because I feel trapped."
2. **Reflect on why**: "It might remind me of a past event where I had no control."
3. **Create an exposure plan**: Work with small steps to face that trigger, building confidence over time.
4. **Update your coping list**: Add a specific method for that trigger, like telling a friend you might leave early if anxiety spikes.

Turning a trigger into an opportunity for growth can lessen its power.

---

10. Working with Acceptance

A big part of handling setbacks is acceptance—not acceptance that the trauma was okay, but acceptance that ups and downs are part of healing. Acceptance might look like:

- **Acknowledging the reality of a setback**: "Yes, I am struggling more right now."
- **Letting go of "should"**: Instead of saying, "I should be cured," accept that healing takes ongoing effort.
- **Treating yourself gently**: Understanding that you may need more rest, comfort, or support at the moment.
- **Avoiding the shame spiral**: Reminding yourself that it is normal to have these waves of symptoms.

Acceptance is not about giving up; it is about not fighting reality and instead channeling your energy into healthy responses.

---

11. Leaning on Your Support Network

When you are in a setback, it is tempting to hide away, but leaning on others can be a powerful way to get through it:

1. **Family or close friends**: Let them know what is happening. If you prefer texts or short visits, say so.
2. **Support groups**: Sharing with people who understand trauma can bring empathy and ideas.
3. **Online communities**: If in-person contact feels too hard, consider a moderated online forum where you can talk about setbacks safely.
4. **Buddy system**: If you have a friend who also deals with anxiety or PTSD, agree to check in on each other during tough times.

People do not always know you need help unless you tell them. A setback can be easier if you do not face it alone.

---

12. Reviewing Your Past Progress

When a setback hits, it is easy to forget how far you have come. Spend a little time recalling:

- **Times you coped well**: What helped you calm down in previous rough patches?
- **Skills you mastered**: Maybe you learned to do grounding exercises or manage nightmares.
- **Challenges you have overcome**: Think of a specific moment that was once too hard but now is easier.
- **Any positive changes**: Even if you feel bad now, maybe you communicate better or have fewer flashbacks than you did months ago.

Remembering your accomplishments can restore hope that this setback is temporary.

---

13. Adjusting Expectations

Healing is not a straight line. If you believed you would never have another flashback or panic attack, a setback might feel like a huge letdown. To handle this:

1. **Expect waves**: Understanding that symptoms might flare up occasionally can soften the blow.

2. **Measure success differently**: Instead of expecting zero panic, look at how quickly you can calm yourself now compared to before.
3. **Set short-term goals**: Focus on feeling a little better each day or doing one helpful thing. Large expectations can be overwhelming when you are in a slump.
4. **Acknowledge partial wins**: Maybe the flashback was strong, but you used your coping skills earlier than last time. That is still a step forward.

Adapting your outlook can prevent extra disappointment when bumps arise.

---

14. Using Self-Soothing Techniques

A setback can bring intense feelings of panic or sadness. Self-soothing is a method to comfort yourself in gentle ways:

- **Touch**: Wrapping up in a soft blanket, hugging a pillow, or giving yourself a light hand massage.
- **Sound**: Listening to calming music, nature sounds, or white noise.
- **Scent**: A mild scent that you find pleasant—like lavender or vanilla—can help calm the mind (if smells are not triggers).
- **Sight**: Looking at photos that make you feel safe or scenes of nature.
- **Taste**: Sipping warm tea or nibbling on a favorite treat, paying attention to its flavor.

These small acts can soothe your system, reminding your brain and body that you are cared for, even if fear or sadness has spiked.

---

15. Thinking Long-Term During a Setback

It is important not to make big life decisions when in a deep setback. Often, intense emotions can cloud judgment. Try:

1. **Delay big choices**: If you are thinking about quitting your job or ending a relationship, see if you can wait until you feel more stable.
2. **Focus on daily coping**: Put your energy into calming and grounding rather than major changes.

3. **Aim for gradual re-balancing**: Once the setback eases, you can reassess your situation with a clearer mind.
4. **Talk to someone you trust**: If a decision cannot wait, get input from a friend or therapist to ensure you are not acting purely from panic.

Thinking long-term means remembering that your current intensity of feelings may soften if you give yourself time.

---

16. Re-Establishing Routines

Setbacks can knock you off your routine. Suddenly, you might sleep at odd hours or skip meals:

- **Gently return to basic routines**: Aim to get back to regular sleeping, eating, and self-care patterns as soon as it feels possible.
- **Use small steps**: If cooking dinner is too much, try a simple sandwich or soup. If a full workout is too draining, do a 5-minute walk.
- **Track progress**: After a few days of consistent routine, you might notice your mood lifting slightly.
- **Reward yourself**: Give yourself a nod of approval when you stick to a basic routine.

Routines act like scaffolding. They help hold you up when everything else feels shaky.

---

17. Finding Meaning in Setbacks

Though setbacks feel distressing, some people discover insights when they look back on them:

- **Identify unhealed parts**: Maybe the setback reveals a memory or trigger you have not addressed fully. This can guide future therapy.
- **Build resilience**: Each time you face a setback and recover, you learn that you can handle these ups and downs.
- **Clarify your needs**: Sometimes the setback happens because you pushed too hard or neglected self-care. This can be a lesson to pace yourself.
- **Strengthen empathy**: Experiencing struggles again can remind you how tough the fight is, deepening compassion for yourself and others.

Seeking meaning does not make the pain vanish, but it can help you use the experience to refine your coping and better understand your healing path.

---

18. When to Seek Immediate Help

While most setbacks can be managed with coping and support, some signs mean you should seek immediate help:

- **Thoughts of self-harm** or a strong desire to end your life.
- **Urges to harm someone else** out of uncontrolled rage or fear.
- **Loss of ability to function** (not eating or drinking for days, or not able to care for yourself at all).
- **Complete detachment from reality** (strong dissociation that does not subside).

Contact a trusted person, call a crisis hotline, or go to the nearest emergency services. You do not have to face a severe crisis alone.

---

19. Encouraging Words for Yourself

During a setback, supportive words can counterbalance panic. Try telling yourself:

- **"This has happened before, and I got through it."**
- **"My feelings are real, but they will not last forever."**
- **"I am not a failure for having a rough time."**
- **"I know some steps to calm down. Let me try one now."**

Treat these words like a lifeline. You can even write them on notes and place them where you will see them often.

Chapter 18: Rebuilding Trust and Bonds

Trauma can harm not only your sense of safety in the world but also the connections you have with other people. You might find it harder to trust loved ones, or you may notice that your relationships feel distant or uneasy after going through a painful event. Rebuilding trust and bonds is possible, though it takes willingness from both you and those around you. In this chapter, we will look at what trust means after trauma, how to heal relationships that have suffered, ways to create new bonds that feel safe, and how to make sure you do not lose yourself in the process. While no one can undo the past, it is possible to learn how to relate to others in healthier, more fulfilling ways.

---

1. Why Trauma Shakes Trust

Trust often rests on the belief that the world is generally predictable and that people close to you will not hurt or abandon you. But trauma—especially if it involves betrayal or an unexpected event—can shatter these assumptions. Some reasons your trust might be shaken include:

1. **Broken promises**: Perhaps someone you relied on did not protect you, or they were the cause of the harm.
2. **Shock of the event**: Even if no one directly hurt you, an extreme situation (like a severe accident) can leave you feeling that nothing is truly safe.
3. **Loss of control**: Trauma can make you feel helpless, which can extend to not feeling safe relying on others.
4. **Self-blame**: Feeling guilty can sometimes twist into believing you cannot trust yourself to judge situations or people correctly.

When trust breaks, it can affect every kind of relationship—family, romantic, friendship, and even your relationship with yourself.

---

2. Recognizing Signs of Trust Struggles

You might not realize at first how deeply trauma has impacted your ability to trust. Some subtle signs:

- **Questioning motives**: You might feel suspicious that people have hidden agendas or are out to trick you.
- **Testing loved ones**: You might create "tests" (consciously or not) to see if people will hurt or abandon you, such as pushing them away to see if they come back.
- **Fear of intimacy**: Getting close—whether emotionally or physically—can feel too risky, leading you to keep a distance.
- **Avoiding reliance on others**: You might do everything yourself because asking for help feels dangerous or humiliating.
- **Jealousy or controlling behaviors**: In romantic relationships, you may feel the need to control or monitor your partner, expecting betrayal at any moment.

These patterns can persist even if logically you know someone is trustworthy. Emotions often overshadow logic when trauma is involved.

---

3. Deciding Whether to Rebuild Trust

Sometimes, the person who broke your trust is the one who caused the trauma (e.g., an abusive family member or partner). In these cases, it might not be safe—or wise—to rebuild trust if the person remains harmful. Key questions:

- **Is the person genuinely remorseful?** If they do not see or admit the harm they caused, trust may be impossible to rebuild.
- **Have they changed or sought help?** If someone is actively working on their behavior—perhaps through therapy or consistent actions—you might consider rebuilding trust.
- **Do you feel safe in their presence?** If your body tenses up or panic overwhelms you, forcing yourself to trust might only harm you further.
- **What do close friends or professionals say?** Sometimes, an outside viewpoint can help you see if a relationship is salvageable or too unsafe.

It is not your duty to forgive or trust everyone who hurt you. Sometimes, walking away protects your well-being. Other times, you might choose to try, with boundaries in place.

---

4. Rebuilding Trust with Family and Friends

If your trauma is linked to events outside your immediate circle, you may still find that relationships feel strained. Loved ones might not understand PTSD, or they might be unsure how to talk to you. Steps to rebuild trust include:

1. **Share your feelings when ready**: Explaining how the trauma affects you can help them see why you act guarded or distant.
2. **Ask for specific support**: If you need people to avoid certain topics or triggers, let them know clearly.
3. **Give small chances**: Trust often grows through small, positive experiences—like letting a friend help you with an errand, then noticing they did not judge you.
4. **Set limits on information**: You do not have to share every detail of your trauma. Reveal only what helps you feel understood and safe.
5. **Express appreciation** (in a way you are comfortable): If someone respects your needs or boundaries, acknowledging their kindness can encourage more supportive behavior.

Rebuilding trust with people who care about you can create a buffer against future stress. Even if it feels awkward at first, these bonds can strengthen over time.

---

5. Healing from Betrayal in Close Relationships

In some cases, the trauma is directly caused by someone you love—a partner, a parent, or a close friend. Healing that kind of betrayal can be more complicated:

- **Acknowledge the betrayal**: Do not downplay or excuse their behavior. Recognize that it damaged you deeply.
- **Seek professional help**: Couples or family therapy can offer a structured environment for airing grievances, learning new communication, and verifying if the person is committed to change.
- **Ask for accountability**: The person who hurt you should be able to take responsibility without shifting blame onto you. They might say, "I was wrong," rather than "I did it because of you."
- **Watch for consistent change**: Rebuilding trust is not about one apology; it requires them showing safer, healthier behavior repeatedly over time.

- **Decide what you need**: Maybe you need an apology, a gesture of goodwill, or an agreement on new boundaries. Clarify these needs if you plan to keep the relationship.

Even if you manage to heal with them, you may still feel echoes of mistrust. That does not mean you are failing—it is a natural response to being deeply hurt.

---

6. Romantic Relationships After Trauma

You might worry that trauma has left you unable to have a healthy romantic connection. While it can be challenging, many people do rebuild loving bonds. Some tips:

1. **Be honest about your triggers**: Early on, you can tell a new partner, "I get anxious if someone raises their voice, so please speak calmly if we argue."
2. **Practice small steps of intimacy**: This might include emotional closeness (sharing feelings) or physical closeness at a pace you can handle.
3. **Learn to self-soothe**: Relying solely on a partner for calm can strain the relationship. Having your own coping methods (breathing, grounding) helps you not feel desperate for their reassurance every time you panic.
4. **Watch for red flags**: If the new partner is dismissive, controlling, or verbally abusive, it is likely not a safe relationship for healing.
5. **Celebrate progress**: When you manage conflict without shutting down or you feel safe enough to share a personal story, notice that as growth.

A patient, understanding partner can be part of the healing process—but be sure not to rush or ignore your need for boundaries.

---

7. Strengthening Bonds Through Communication

Whether you are trying to reconnect with family, friends, or a partner, open communication can mend the gaps trauma left behind. Some communication skills:

- **Use "I" statements**: Say, "I feel anxious when the topic of my accident is brought up suddenly," rather than "You always upset me."

- **Be specific**: Instead of saying, "I'm stressed," say, "When there are loud noises, I feel panicked because it reminds me of what happened."
- **Listen in return**: Ask them how they feel, too. Sometimes trauma survivors get so focused on their own fear that they forget others might have feelings about the changes in your relationship.
- **Check for understanding**: After explaining something, you might gently ask, "Does that make sense? Do you have any questions about what I said?"
- **Talk about future plans**: Planning small events or shared activities can help you both look forward instead of being stuck in the past.

Good communication does not fix everything overnight, but it sets a foundation for trust to grow, as each person feels heard and respected.

---

8. Building Trust with Yourself

Trauma can also destroy your self-trust. You might feel:

- **Guilty or ashamed**: Blaming yourself for not preventing the event.
- **Doubtful of your intuition**: If you sensed something was wrong but did not act, you might think your judgment is unreliable.
- **Afraid to make decisions**: Worrying you will fail or cause more harm.

Rebuilding self-trust involves:

1. **Rewriting self-blame**: Remind yourself that you had limited power, and the responsibility belongs to the harmful situation or person, not you.
2. **Taking small risks**: Trying new hobbies or making minor decisions (like picking a new recipe) can slowly rebuild confidence in your choices.
3. **Monitoring self-talk**: Replace thoughts like "I always mess up" with "I am learning and growing. Mistakes are part of that."
4. **Noticing successes**: Even small wins—like managing a trigger without panicking as much—show you can trust your ability to cope.

As you begin trusting your own judgment again, it becomes easier to trust others in a measured, healthy way.

---

9. Navigating Boundaries

Healing from trauma often involves clarifying your boundaries—what you need to feel safe and comfortable:

1. **Identify your limits**: Maybe you cannot handle discussing certain events late at night, or you need personal space if someone raises their voice.
2. **Communicate boundaries**: Let people know clearly, "I don't want to talk about that subject," or "I need a break if we argue."
3. **Enforce consequences**: If someone repeatedly violates your boundaries, step away or end the conversation. This is not mean; it is self-protection.
4. **Adjust boundaries as you grow**: Over time, you might find you can handle more. Or you might discover you need stricter boundaries with certain people.

Boundaries do not block intimacy; they create a framework that keeps trust from being undermined by disrespect or misunderstanding.

---

10. Group Activities and Community Connection

Part of rebuilding trust involves stepping into social or communal settings. This might be:

- **Support groups**: Meeting others who have gone through similar traumas can help you see you are not alone, and you can learn from each other's experiences.
- **Volunteering**: Helping a local charity or community project can gently remind you that people can be kind and appreciative, which can rebuild a sense of shared humanity.
- **Hobby clubs or classes**: Joining a group activity (like a book club, dance class, or art workshop) can shift focus away from fear and toward shared interests.
- **Community events**: Attending local gatherings in small steps—maybe staying for just 20 minutes at first—can expand your comfort zone.

Being around others in a structured environment can challenge the notion that all people are dangerous. Over time, you may find your social confidence returning.

11. Self-Reflection and Journaling for Trust Growth

Keeping track of your thoughts and feelings about trust can help you spot patterns and progress:

- **Journal triggers**: If a friend's harmless question made you angry or suspicious, write down why you felt that way. Maybe it reminded you of something from the past.
- **Note positive interactions**: Document when someone supported you or respected a boundary. This helps challenge the idea that "no one is trustworthy."
- **Reflect on your own actions**: If you lashed out or withdrew, ask yourself what fear might have driven that reaction.
- **Plan for next time**: If a situation arises again, how could you respond differently?

Self-reflection fosters a deeper understanding of why you feel mistrust and how to slowly shift toward healthier connections.

---

12. Taking Slow Steps Toward Intimacy

If physical or emotional closeness triggers fear (common in trauma survivors), you can build comfort through gradual exposure to safe, supportive people:

1. **Safe touch**: If hugging is scary, start with a brief, gentle handshake or let someone place a hand on your shoulder for a second. Increase as you feel more at ease.
2. **Eye contact**: Holding eye contact can feel very intimate. If it is too intense, practice shorter glances or do it only with a person you trust.
3. **Emotional sharing**: Instead of revealing deep trauma details, start by sharing smaller personal experiences or feelings to gauge the other person's response.
4. **Direct reassurance**: It can help to hear a friend or partner say, "You can tell me if this is too much," or "We can slow down if you feel uncomfortable."

Over time, if the person consistently respects your pace, your body and mind can learn that closeness does not always mean danger.

13. Handling Fear of Loss or Abandonment

Trauma can also create a fear of losing people you love. You might cling too tightly or avoid closeness to prevent the pain of potential loss. Ways to manage this include:

- **Acknowledge the fear**: Recognize that part of you is scared of being left behind or hurt again.
- **Build personal resilience**: The stronger and more self-reliant you feel, the less likely you are to panic about someone leaving.
- **Open communication**: If you worry a friend or partner will go away, talk about it gently. They may reassure you or discuss how they handle conflict.
- **Therapy around abandonment**: A counselor can help you process past losses or betrayals so you do not project them onto your current relationships.

The aim is not to ignore your fear but to handle it in ways that allow closeness without suffocating the other person or sabotaging the bond.

14. Recognizing Trust Milestones

As you work on rebuilding trust and bonds, you might see small milestones:

- **A friend respects a boundary**: You asked them not to bring up a painful topic, and they follow through.
- **You express vulnerability**: You share a personal fear, and the person responds supportively instead of judging you.
- **You rely on someone else**: Maybe you let a neighbor help carry groceries, and it went fine.
- **You notice less tension**: Over time, you might realize you are not as jumpy or suspicious around people you know well.

Recognizing these moments helps you see that trust can grow bit by bit. They show you that progress is happening, even if larger challenges remain.

15. Coping with Setbacks in Trust

Just like with personal healing, relationship trust can face setbacks. For instance, you might have a flashback that makes you question everyone around you, or a misunderstanding might trigger your old fears. To handle these setbacks:

1. **Pause and reflect**: Ask yourself whether the current situation truly mirrors past harm or if your trauma responses might be magnifying it.
2. **Communicate**: If possible, tell the person involved, "I'm feeling triggered because of my past experiences. I need some reassurance or space right now."
3. **Use coping strategies**: Grounding exercises or self-talk can calm your initial panic so you can see the situation more clearly.
4. **Get professional help if needed**: A therapist can mediate conflicts or help you separate past trauma from present reality.
5. **Re-commit to trust-building**: After the immediate flare-up settles, return to the small steps that previously helped you.

A setback in trust does not mean you have to start from scratch. You can learn from it and move forward again.

---

16. Dealing with People Who Do Not Understand

Some individuals might not understand why you are cautious or distant. They may say unhelpful things like:

- **"Just get over it!"**
- **"Why do you still not trust me?"**
- **"That happened ages ago—stop living in the past."**

In these cases:

- **Explain briefly if you wish**: "I'm still working through effects of what happened, so it will take time."
- **Set boundaries**: If they keep dismissing you, limit contact or discussions about your trauma.
- **Seek understanding elsewhere**: Focus on people who respect your situation.

- **Avoid internalizing ignorance**: Their lack of empathy is about them, not a reflection of you.

You do not need everyone's approval. What matters is having a supportive circle that honors your feelings and growth pace.

---

17. Collective Healing in Families

When trauma affects a family—maybe a natural disaster or a shared loss—everyone might struggle with trust in different ways. Possible family steps:

1. **Family therapy**: A counselor can help each member express their experience and respect each other's coping styles.
2. **Joint activities**: Doing safe, positive projects or recreation together can rebuild a sense of unity.
3. **Honest conversations**: Encourage each person to share how the trauma changed them, and what they need from others.
4. **Respect individual timelines**: Some family members may recover faster than others. Pushing someone to "move on" can harm trust further.
5. **Agree on conflict rules**: For example, no yelling or name-calling if arguments happen. This fosters a safer environment.

Families can either fracture or grow closer after trauma, and the difference often lies in whether everyone is willing to learn and communicate.

---

18. Spiritual or Faith-Based Trust

If faith or spirituality was part of your life before trauma, you might feel your trust in a higher power or your spiritual community is shaken. Rebuilding that aspect can involve:

- **Talking to faith leaders**: A trusted pastor, rabbi, imam, or spiritual mentor might offer guidance on questions about suffering and safety.
- **Joining supportive groups**: Some faith communities have small groups specifically for grief or trauma healing.
- **Exploring personal reflection**: Meditation, prayer, or reading spiritual texts might help you find new understanding of how trust fits into your belief system.

- **Allowing doubt**: It is normal to question beliefs after trauma. Sometimes, working through these doubts with openness leads to a deeper, more nuanced faith or spiritual practice.

This part is highly personal. Some find comfort and renewed trust in their spiritual beliefs, while others choose a different path. Both are valid.

---

19. The Role of Time in Rebuilding Trust

You may feel impatient, wishing you could quickly trust again and feel close to people. But trust is not a quick fix:

1. **Patience is key**: Expecting immediate results can lead to frustration. Healing from deep wounds often takes months or years.
2. **Consistent positive experiences**: Each supportive conversation or respectful action from others gradually rewrites the narrative that "people always hurt me."
3. **Ongoing self-work**: Your own triggers and fears will likely resurface from time to time, requiring continued self-compassion and coping methods.

Time alone does not heal, but consistent, caring actions over time do.

Chapter 19: Keeping Problems from Returning

Healing from trauma or PTSD does not always follow a tidy path. You may have gone through therapy, learned coping skills, rebuilt trust in yourself or others, and found stability. Yet you might still wonder, "How do I ensure these problems do not come back in full force? What if I fall into old habits?" This concern is normal. Maintenance—making sure that progress sticks—is a big part of living with trauma's effects over the long term. In this chapter, we will look at relapse prevention strategies: how to catch early warning signs, the role of continued self-care, ways to adapt your methods as life changes, and how to handle those moments when problems begin to creep back in.

1. What Does "Keeping Problems from Returning" Mean?

After significant progress, you might no longer experience constant flashbacks or daily panic. However, "keeping problems from returning" does not imply you will never feel anxious or triggered again. Rather, it means:

- **Recognizing early signs** that your symptoms might be rising.
- **Taking prompt action** to manage or reduce those symptoms before they become overwhelming.
- **Sustaining healthy routines** and coping strategies instead of letting them slip away when you start feeling better.
- **Accepting that small setbacks can happen** but can be kept from turning into a full-blown crisis.

In essence, it is a lifestyle approach—continuing to care for your mental health so you remain as stable and resilient as possible.

2. Maintaining Self-Awareness

One of the biggest pitfalls after you feel better is forgetting to pay attention to your emotional health. Signs that trouble might be returning include:

- **Trouble sleeping**: Old patterns of insomnia or nightmares creeping back in.

- **Heightened irritability**: Snapping at people more than usual or feeling tension simmer all day.
- **Avoidance returning**: You start skipping social events, ignoring calls, or avoiding certain places again.
- **Negative self-talk**: Thoughts like "I'm worthless," "I can't do anything right," or "Nobody cares" reemerge.
- **Physical symptoms**: Headaches, stomachaches, or muscle pain that show stress is building.

By keeping track of these subtle signals—perhaps in a journal or mental checklist—you can step in early to prevent a slide back into severe symptoms.

3. Regular Check-Ins and Tune-Ups

Even if you no longer see a therapist weekly, scheduling periodic check-ins can help:

1. **Therapy tune-ups**: Maybe see your counselor once a month or every few months to discuss any new concerns or changes.
2. **Support group visits**: Dropping into a group session from time to time can remind you of coping skills and let you share experiences with others.
3. **Mental health "self-check"**: Every Sunday, for instance, you might reflect on how you felt that week, any triggers faced, and whether you used your coping tools effectively.
4. **Chat with a trusted friend**: Sometimes, a friend who knows your journey well can ask, "How are you, really?" and help you see issues you might miss.

These check-ins act as preventive maintenance, like taking a car for regular servicing rather than waiting for it to break down.

4. Guarding Against Complacency

When life becomes calmer, it is natural to want to stop thinking about trauma-related issues. While rest from intense focus is good, letting all your healthy habits slide can leave you unprepared if triggers appear. Examples of complacency:

- **Quitting coping methods**: No longer doing grounding exercises or relaxation because "I feel fine now."
- **Ignoring stress**: Letting small worries build up instead of addressing them.
- **Skipping healthy routines**: Abandoning the regular sleep schedule or healthy eating habits that once helped you.
- **Cutting off support**: Stopping therapy too soon or dropping contact with supportive friends.

Staying balanced does not mean you have to dwell on trauma every day, but it does mean keeping up the routines and skills that helped stabilize you in the first place.

5. Updating Coping Skills as Life Changes

The strategies that worked at one stage might need tweaking later. Maybe you have a new job, a different living situation, or changed health conditions. Adapting coping methods is key:

1. **Reevaluate triggers**: A move to a bustling city might trigger noise-based anxiety, needing different grounding skills than you needed before.
2. **Add new tools**: If you started practicing yoga and found it helpful, incorporate it more often. Or if you discovered an online support community, integrate it into your routine.
3. **Discard methods that no longer fit**: A coping method might have lost its effectiveness or become impractical. That is okay—replace it with something else.
4. **Stay open to learning**: Continued reading, occasional workshops, or new therapy techniques can refresh your approach.

Flexibility is crucial because life rarely stays the same. A fluid coping plan can handle these shifts without losing stability.

6. Building a Sustainable Lifestyle

Keeping problems from returning is easier when your overall life pattern supports mental well-being. Some pillars of a sustainable lifestyle include:

- **Consistent sleep schedule**: Aim for enough rest each night. Chronic fatigue weakens your resilience to stress.
- **Reasonable workload**: Overcommitting at work or school can lead to burnout, making you vulnerable to relapse.
- **Balanced nutrition**: Not perfection, but steady, nourishing meals that keep your body fueled.
- **Physical activity**: Gentle exercise or walks can help regulate stress hormones.
- **Time for joy**: Hobbies, music, art, or any activity that sparks a sense of fun or creativity keeps negativity from dominating.
- **Social connections**: Maintaining at least a few relationships where you feel safe and accepted.

When these elements form the backbone of your daily life, you have a stronger buffer against stress.

---

7. Using Early Intervention Plans

An early intervention plan details exactly what you will do if you spot signs of a relapse. It might include:

1. **Warning signs**: A list of thoughts, feelings, or behaviors that indicate trouble is brewing.
2. **Immediate actions**: Coping skills you will use right away—like taking a short walk, doing a grounding exercise, or calling a trusted friend.
3. **Support contacts**: Names and phone numbers of people (friends, crisis lines, mental health professionals) you can reach out to if the situation worsens.
4. **Short-term adjustments**: For instance, "If I have trouble sleeping three nights in a row, I will cut back on social media and caffeine, and try a relaxing bedtime routine."
5. **Emergency steps**: If it escalates, you might have a plan to check into a mental health clinic or call a counselor for an urgent appointment.

Review this plan occasionally and update it as your life changes.

---

8. Staying Mindful of Relationships

Relationships can play a big role in relapse prevention—both positively and negatively:

- **Positive**: Encouraging friends or a supportive partner can notice if you seem off-balance and gently mention it, giving you a chance to address issues early.
- **Negative**: Toxic or draining relationships can push you toward exhaustion or heightened stress, making old symptoms resurface.
- **Boundaries**: Maintaining clear boundaries keeps relationships healthy and prevents over-involvement or emotional burnout.
- **Ongoing communication**: Let people close to you know that if they see certain changes in your behavior—withdrawal, anger, or panic—they can kindly bring it to your attention.

The people you surround yourself with can be an early warning system or a source of strain, so choose carefully.

---

9. Creating Meaning and Purpose

Trauma can rob you of a sense of purpose. Finding or rediscovering meaning in life can protect against slipping back:

1. **Volunteering**: Helping others can remind you that you have value and can make a difference.
2. **Creative pursuits**: Arts, crafts, writing, or music can channel emotions into a productive outlet.
3. **Personal projects**: This could be learning a new skill or working toward a meaningful goal like finishing a degree.
4. **Spiritual or philosophical exploration**: Some people find renewed purpose in faith or introspection.

Having something that fuels hope and direction can act as a buffer when old trauma feelings threaten to resurface.

---

10. Addressing Physical Health

Physical health and mental health are closely connected. Ignoring bodily concerns can lead to a decline in emotional well-being:

- **Attend regular check-ups**: Untreated medical issues can create chronic stress, fueling emotional instability.
- **Exercise in moderation**: Even a little bit of daily movement can reduce tension and regulate mood.
- **Manage chronic pain** if present: Pain can trigger irritability and anxiety, so proper treatment or pain management strategies help keep stress lower.
- **Limit harmful substances**: Excessive alcohol or recreational drug use can worsen PTSD symptoms or disrupt coping mechanisms.

A strong body can lend stability to a healing mind. They do not have to be perfect, but consistent care helps.

---

11. Staying Open to New Phases of Healing

Sometimes, you might think you have resolved your trauma fully, only to uncover deeper layers later. This does not mean you are going backward:

- **Different life stages** (e.g., marriage, parenthood, a new job) can activate old emotions.
- **Additional therapies** like trauma-informed yoga, EMDR, or group counseling might be helpful at a new stage.
- **Evolving perspective**: As you grow older, you might interpret your past differently and need fresh ways to process it.

Staying open means you do not panic when new insights or feelings arise; you treat them as another opportunity to refine your healing approach.

---

12. Dealing with Unforeseen Crises

Sometimes life throws major stressors your way—serious illness, job loss, relationship breakups—that are not directly about the trauma but can weaken your emotional defenses. In these crises:

1. **Return to basics**: Lean on the coping skills you learned early in your trauma healing, like grounding exercises or reaching out for support.
2. **Seek temporary professional help**: Even a few sessions with a therapist can keep a crisis from reigniting severe PTSD symptoms.
3. **Mobilize your support system**: Let friends or family know you are in a tough spot, so they can provide emotional or practical help.
4. **Set boundaries on new stress**: If possible, postpone non-urgent commitments until you feel more stable.

Handling big life changes with the same care you used for trauma recovery lowers the chance of a full relapse.

---

13. The Role of Forgiveness and Acceptance

For some people, part of preventing a recurrence of trauma symptoms involves ongoing work around forgiveness—whether that is forgiving those who caused the harm, or forgiving yourself for actions or inactions during the traumatic period. However:

- **Forgiveness is personal**: You do not owe it to anyone if it does not serve your healing.
- **Acceptance is not agreement**: Accepting that the trauma happened and cannot be changed helps you move forward. It does not mean you think it was okay.
- **Self-forgiveness**: Blaming yourself drains energy you could use to maintain well-being. Recognizing your limits at the time and letting go of guilt can keep stress from piling up again.

If these themes continue to trouble you, therapy can provide a structured space to explore them without pressuring yourself.

---

14. Acknowledging Progress Along the Way

When your symptoms are less intense and your daily life is more stable, it can be easy to forget how far you have come. Recognizing your growth keeps you motivated:

1. **Keep a "pride list"**: Note things you can now do that were once impossible—like visiting a crowded store, sleeping without nightmares, or maintaining a calm conversation during conflict.
2. **Share achievements**: Telling a friend or counselor about your progress can help solidify the positive feeling.
3. **Reflect in a journal**: Write about the differences in your life compared to a year ago. You may see a surprising number of positive changes.

These affirmations remind you that you possess the resilience to keep problems at bay. They also give you a confidence boost if new challenges arise.

---

15. Understanding That Relapse Is Not Failure

Even with all these precautions, you might still have periods when symptoms surge. This is not a failure; it is part of a long-term journey. If a relapse happens:

- **Use your early intervention plan**: Tackle it as soon as you notice.
- **Avoid harsh self-criticism**: Self-blame can worsen the relapse. Instead, treat it as a challenge you are equipped to handle.
- **Seek extra support**: Sometimes, a short burst of therapy or more frequent group meetings is enough to get you back on track.
- **Learn from the event**: Ask, "What triggered this relapse? What can I change or add to my plan to reduce the chance of it happening again?"
- **Revisit old coping tools**: You might remember something that helped you before—like writing letters you never send, or doing creative projects to process feelings.

Relapse does not erase your progress; it just calls for renewed effort to stabilize and move forward once more.

---

16. Balancing Hope and Realism

Staying free from major PTSD problems is easier if you strike a balance between optimism and realism:

- **Optimism**: You can hope to lead a fulfilling life, with trauma playing a smaller role. Believe that you have grown and can keep growing.

- **Realism**: Acknowledge that triggers might still appear, and you may always need some coping strategies in place.
- **Healthy viewpoint**: It is not about ignoring the past but about being prepared to manage it if it surfaces again.

This balanced mindset reduces shock if difficulties reappear and helps you appreciate the better days without fear that it is "too good to last."

---

17. Ongoing Self-Care as Prevention

We have covered the importance of routines, coping skills, and relationships. These all feed into daily self-care, which acts like a shield against relapse:

- **Mindful mornings**: Start each day with a gentle routine or quick mental check, so you do not rush into stress.
- **Regular breaks**: Even on busy days, micro-pauses to stretch, breathe, or snack can keep stress from boiling over.
- **Winding down at night**: A bedtime routine—like reading or listening to calming sounds—helps your brain shift out of worry mode.
- **Staying hydrated and fed**: Skipping water or meals can spike anxiety or irritability.
- **Plan enjoyable moments**: Scheduling small rewards or relaxing activities prevents life from becoming all chores and no pleasure.

In short, consistent self-care is the daily maintenance that keeps your mental health engine running smoothly.

---

18. Helping Others While Protecting Yourself

As you become more stable, you might feel drawn to help others facing trauma. This can be meaningful, but also risky if you give too much:

1. **Share your story selectively**: Decide when and how much to disclose about your journey.
2. **Set limits**: If someone's needs are overwhelming you, it is okay to direct them to professional resources or say you must step back.

3. **Use peer support responsibly**: Listening to others' trauma can trigger your own memories. Notice if your anxiety spikes and practice self-care.
4. **Remember you are not a therapist**: Unless you are trained, do not carry the burden of someone else's deep trauma. Encourage them to seek professional help when needed.

Being supportive is rewarding, but keep your own mental health protected so you do not slip back into struggle yourself.

---

19. Periodic Reinvention

Life changes, and so do you. Sometimes you might find yourself at a new crossroads—like changing careers, moving to a new place, or embracing a new hobby. Approach these changes with the same mindfulness you use for PTSD:

- **Expect a learning curve**: New settings can trigger old fears or create new stressors.
- **Apply your coping framework**: If you start feeling unsettled, check your early intervention plan, practice grounding, or talk to your support network.
- **Acknowledge growth**: Reinvention can be a sign that you have moved past old barriers, so let yourself feel proud, but remain watchful for potential triggers.
- **Stay flexible**: If a new path proves too overwhelming, break it into smaller steps or reconsider if it is right for you.

Growth and change are natural parts of life. They do not have to threaten your stability if you remain adaptable and well-prepared.

Chapter 20: Looking Ahead with Hope

As you reach this final chapter, it may be helpful to pause and notice how much you have learned about Post-Traumatic Stress Disorder (PTSD) and its impact on daily life. We have covered a wide range of topics—understanding what trauma is, handling painful memories, developing everyday strategies for stress, and keeping yourself steady after making progress. This last chapter is about looking ahead. It is not a promise that life will be perfect, but an invitation to consider what hope can look like, even when you still carry the weight of difficult experiences.

Trauma can cast long shadows, yet you have discovered that change is possible. Hope does not mean you will never feel scared or hurt again. It means you can hold onto the truth that healing is real, that positive steps are in your reach, and that your life can include rich, meaningful experiences no matter what happened in the past. Here, we will explore what it means to move forward with optimism, how to plan for a future shaped more by your strengths than by the trauma, and how to encourage hope both for yourself and possibly for others who are going through something similar.

1. What Hope Really Means After Trauma

In everyday talk, "hope" might sound like a simple wish for good things to come. But when dealing with PTSD, hope takes on a deeper meaning:

1. **Recognizing growth**: You have developed coping skills, practiced setting boundaries, and found ways to handle triggers. These are signs you can adapt and strengthen yourself further.
2. **Allowing emotional range**: Hope does not push away sadness, anger, or fear. Instead, it makes room for new feelings like relief, calm, and even happiness.
3. **Seeing potential in small changes**: You do not need a huge turning point to have hope. Each small step you take is a reminder that you are not stuck.
4. **Accepting that life can hold both pain and promise**: Hope acknowledges that the trauma did happen and might still affect you, yet it does not have to dictate every aspect of your future.

Hope stands alongside honesty about lingering trauma. It is a choice to keep going, to continue learning, and to trust that each day can bring a bit more clarity or peace.

---

2. Reviewing Your Achievements and Strengths

Before you look forward, it can help to look back at how far you have come. Even if you still have moments of anxiety or difficulties with trust, you likely have some wins to acknowledge:

- **Coping Skills Learned**: Perhaps you found grounding exercises effective or discovered that talking with a friend soothes your nerves.
- **Triggers Managed**: You may have identified certain smells, sounds, or scenarios that trigger flashbacks, and learned how to lower their power.
- **Healthier Boundaries**: In personal or work relationships, you might have practiced saying "no" or explaining your needs clearly, protecting yourself from unnecessary stress.
- **Reduced Avoidance**: If you used to avoid certain places or conversations, maybe you have taken steps—like visiting a location briefly or gradually discussing tough memories with a safe person.
- **Moments of Joy**: There may have been days or hours when you felt calm, connected, or even happy. Noticing these experiences can reinforce the idea that life is not all shadow.

Recognizing your achievements is not about ignoring ongoing struggles. It is about showing yourself that change is real, which can fuel hope for continued growth.

---

3. Imagining Your Future

After trauma, it can be scary or overwhelming to think about the future. You might fear disappointment or worry about triggers waiting around the corner. But imagining a tomorrow that is broader than your pain can help you see that you still have choices:

1. **Picture small goals**: Sometimes, big dreams feel impossible. Start with a modest vision—maybe wanting a stable daily routine, stronger friendships, or a newfound hobby.

2. **Allow flexible thinking**: Your future might not be a single grand plan but a series of evolving interests and directions. That is normal and healthy.
3. **Stay open to new experiences**: Even if you tried something once and it triggered you, there might be another way or time to approach it without the same stress.
4. **Consider helping others**: Some people find hope by volunteering, sharing their recovery insights, or just being a kind friend to someone else going through difficulties.

Visualizing the future does not mean forcing yourself to be endlessly positive. It means making space for possibilities that exist beyond trauma.

---

4. Planning for Setbacks

Having hope does not exclude the reality that PTSD symptoms may flare up again. In fact, hope is stronger when you include a plan for potential setbacks:

- **Keep your early warning signs in mind**: You have likely identified signs that trouble might be brewing. Spot them early and use your coping plan.
- **Regular tune-ups**: Think of hope as something that grows when nurtured. Continuing therapy check-ins or peer support helps keep your coping tools sharp.
- **Honest self-talk**: If you feel old fears returning, remind yourself, "I have handled this before. I can manage it now."
- **Adjust as you grow**: If a new job or living situation triggers different stresses, adapt your prevention plan. Keep refining how you respond to triggers in fresh contexts.

Anticipating setbacks might feel like admitting defeat, but it is actually a sign of strength. You are being realistic, which helps you move through difficulties with less fear.

---

5. Allowing Yourself to Dream Again

Trauma can narrow your vision, making it hard to dream about the life you truly want. Reconnecting with hope may involve daring to dream, even if softly:

1. **Recall old interests**: Were there activities or fields you used to be curious about before trauma took over? Can you revisit them now, in small steps?
2. **Try new directions**: Maybe you have never tried painting or short weekend trips. Testing these waters can spark a sense of possibility.
3. **Look for role models**: Others who have grown past their trauma might show you that healing can lead to meaningful projects, friendships, or achievements you never considered.
4. **Practice stepping out of the comfort zone**: Hope is nurtured when you see yourself handle something a bit uncertain and survive it, or even enjoy it.

Dreaming is not naive if you also keep your boundaries and coping strategies in place. It is about welcoming life's potential without pretending trauma did not happen.

6. Balancing Acceptance with Hope

Acceptance and hope might seem like opposites. Acceptance could imply settling, while hope suggests aiming for something better. But they can support each other:

- **Accepting what happened**: Acknowledging that the trauma was real and shaped part of who you are.
- **Accepting ongoing impact**: Recognizing that certain triggers or sensitivities might remain.
- **Holding hope for better management**: You may never be entirely free of triggers, but you can trust that your response to them can keep improving.
- **Letting acceptance free you**: Once you stop fighting the fact that trauma changed some aspects of your life, you can pour energy into building new strengths and joys.

In that balance, you can find peace in where you are now, while still believing in and working toward further growth.

7. Sustaining Healthy Connections

Hope is often fueled by relationships that affirm your worth and remind you that you are not alone:

1. **Keep nurturing existing bonds**: If you have supportive friends, family, or a partner, continue honest communication and share your progress or concerns.
2. **Reach out when lonely**: Part of looking ahead is knowing you do not have to face triggers in isolation. A quick text or call can break the sense of being alone in your struggle.
3. **Consider new communities**: If old circles do not support your healing, explore new groups—social clubs, spiritual communities, or peer support settings.
4. **Respect your boundaries**: Not everyone is safe or kind, so keep trusting your instincts about who deserves your time and openness.

Healthy connections can shine a light on hopeful possibilities, reminding you that caring people exist and that closeness can be safe and rewarding.

---

8. Contributing to Others' Well-Being

As you gain stability, you might look for ways to help people who are still in earlier stages of trauma recovery. This can reinforce your own hope:

- **Offer gentle advice**: If a friend is going through something similar, you can share what coping skills worked for you.
- **Volunteer in mental health or social services**: Some organizations welcome peers who have "been there" to offer support or simply a listening ear.
- **Engage in positive storytelling**: When appropriate, sharing your journey—where you started and where you are now—can give others realistic hope.
- **Respect your limits**: Helping others should not push you back into distress. If you feel overloaded, scale back and care for yourself first.

Giving to others often brings perspective, reinforcing that your experiences, while painful, have forged empathy and resilience that can benefit not only you but also those around you.

---

9. Continuing Personal Growth

Trauma may have taught you about your own strength, but there is always more to discover. Continuing personal growth might include:

1. **Exploring new interests**: Whether it is learning an instrument, studying a language, or taking small online courses, fresh learning can keep you feeling engaged with the world.
2. **Trying healthier challenges**: Maybe you want to practice public speaking in a supportive group or try a mild adventure like a nature walk with friends. Facing controlled challenges can expand your sense of capability.
3. **Reflecting on values**: Trauma can change what matters to you. Clarify what you now value—maybe it is compassion, honesty, creativity—and let that guide future choices.
4. **Allowing change in identity**: You might no longer identify purely as a "trauma survivor." Perhaps you see yourself as an artist, a helper, a parent, or a friend. Embrace those evolving roles.

Personal growth is not about ignoring trauma but about not letting it remain the main or only part of your life story.

---

10. Small Moments of Beauty

In the wake of trauma, noticing small wonders in everyday life can be a powerful form of hope:

- **Observing nature**: Watching a sunrise, listening to birds, or tending a small plant can remind you of renewal.
- **Engaging your senses**: Really taste your food, feel the texture of a cozy blanket, or smell a light fragrance. These mindful acts root you in a peaceful present, instead of past fear.
- **Seeking art or music**: A song that speaks to your experience or a painting that inspires calm can feed a sense of connection and gratitude.

Finding beauty in small things does not erase trauma, but it stretches your capacity to feel and notice goodness.

---

11. Handling Uncertain Times

The world is not always predictable. Global events, natural disasters, or community tensions can stir up fear, especially if they echo aspects of your trauma. Facing uncertainty with hope might involve:

- **Keeping a stable routine**: Even if the news is unsettling, cling to simple habits—wake-up times, meal patterns, or bedtime rituals.
- **Limiting media exposure**: Constantly hearing about stressful events can intensify anxiety. Balancing staying informed with maintaining emotional balance helps.
- **Looking for acts of kindness**: In tough times, people often help each other. Paying attention to kindness in the midst of chaos can remind you that not everything is dangerous.
- **Sharing concerns**: If you have a therapist or supportive friend, talk about how large-scale events affect your sense of safety. Possibly set up extra check-ins.

Hope does not deny global problems. It acknowledges them while taking steps to protect your inner well-being.

---

12. Marking Transitions

As you move forward, you might experience transitions that signal shifts in your life: finishing a therapy program, moving to a new place, or celebrating a birthday that once felt overshadowed by trauma anniversaries. Some ways to mark these transitions:

1. **Symbolic gestures**: Writing a letter to your past self and then storing it or tearing it up, whichever feels freeing.
2. **Simple ceremonies**: Lighting a candle or planting a flower can signify entering a new phase.
3. **Talking to loved ones**: Share with a close friend or family member what this transition means to you.
4. **Creating a memory box**: If you have objects or notes linked to your healing, keep them in a box to remind yourself of how you progressed.

Though you might not use the word "celebrate" or "journey," you can still acknowledge the significance of moving into a healthier chapter of life.

13. Reinforcing Positive Self-View

Trauma can leave you feeling unworthy or permanently damaged. Cultivating a better sense of self can sustain hope:

- **Practice affirmations**: Gentle statements like, "I am capable of learning and adapting," or "I am allowed to find peace."
- **Accept imperfections**: Everyone has flaws. Recognizing them without harsh judgment allows you to focus on what you can improve.
- **Remember your resilience**: Whenever you handle a trigger or solve a stressful problem, note how that shows your ability to cope.
- **Seek feedback from those who care**: Sometimes hearing a friend say, "You have such kindness," or "You've come so far," can challenge a negative self-image.

Over time, these positive messages can reshape your sense of self, reminding you that PTSD is a part of your story, not your entire identity.

14. Spreading Hope in Your Environment

If you are feeling steadier, you can influence your environment to be calmer or more uplifting:

- **Keep calming items visible**: A small reminder like a photograph of nature or an inspiring quote can ground you when you feel stressed.
- **Arrange supportive spaces**: If possible, organize your living area to include a quiet corner or bring in gentle scents or soothing lighting.
- **Model calm responses**: People around you might absorb some of your steadiness. When conflict arises, responding calmly can help them do the same.
- **Encourage open discussion**: If you have family or roommates, being open about your self-care routines or boundaries can create a healthier household dynamic.

These changes, though small, make it easier to maintain hope and keep trauma from dominating your daily life.

15. Blending Healing with Normal Challenges

Even as you heal, you might face regular life stresses like paying bills, dealing with busy schedules, or routine arguments with loved ones. The presence of these normal challenges does not mean your trauma healing is derailed. It means:

1. **You are living a fuller life**: Experiencing typical ups and downs is part of being human, not just a trauma survivor.
2. **Use the same coping methods**: Whether you are anxious about finances or a flashback, you can use grounding, breathing, or support-seeking.
3. **Accept imperfection**: Everyone faces some stress in life. Your goal is not to eliminate all problems, but to respond to them without letting trauma patterns take over.
4. **Check your perspective**: Sometimes, a normal issue might feel huge if it activates old fears. Step back and see if it is truly a severe crisis or just life being life.

When you realize you are managing regular challenges alongside past trauma, it can strengthen your sense of hope and autonomy.

---

16. Writing Your Next Chapter

Not using the word "journey," but you can still consider your life story as something you are shaping every day. Trauma might have written some early chapters, but you have the pen now:

- **Identify themes**: Perhaps resilience, empathy, or personal growth appear in your life story. Highlight those themes in your actions and choices.
- **Edit negative scripts**: If your mind says, "I can't trust anyone," you can rewrite it to, "I'm learning who and how to trust safely."
- **Add new experiences**: Trying a new activity, meeting different people, or exploring personal goals can expand your life story beyond the past event.
- **Stay open to surprises**: You do not need a rigid plan for how your future must unfold. Keep a curious attitude, letting good things unfold in unexpected ways.

Seeing life as an evolving story helps you remain hopeful that tomorrow can hold developments you have not yet imagined.

---

17. Encouraging Hope in Others

If you have grown stronger in your coping, you might gently inspire hope in those who see no light at the end of their struggles. Without overstepping:

1. **Share experiences mindfully**: Mention that you also believed things would never get better, yet you found small steps that helped.
2. **Suggest resources**: If you know of good therapists, support lines, or websites, you can share that information.
3. **Offer listening**: Sometimes, the best gift is calm presence—listening without judgment or rushing to fix.
4. **Respect their path**: Understand that each person's growth pace is different. Pressuring them to hurry can backfire.

By showing that healing is possible, you reinforce your own hope and provide a spark for someone else.

---

18. Renewing Hope Over Time

Hope is not a static thing you either have or do not have. It can flicker and fade, then surge again. To renew hope:

1. **Engage in uplifting reading or media**: Sometimes, a memoir of someone who overcame adversity, or an inspiring documentary, can remind you that resilience is real.
2. **Talk to a mentor or close friend**: Hearing them reflect on your growth can spark hope. They might see progress you overlook.
3. **Practice gratitude**: Listing people or moments you appreciate can show that, even with lingering pain, life holds goodness.
4. **Track mental health patterns**: Notice if certain times of year (like anniversaries) or stress points reduce your hope. Prepare extra self-care or professional help before those periods.

Hope is an active choice—a flame you tend. When it dims, gentle actions can reignite it.

Conclusion

Looking ahead with hope after trauma is not about dismissing the hardships you have faced. It is about understanding that, while your past remains part of you, it does not have to define all of your tomorrows. Through the chapters of this book, you have explored the nature of PTSD, recognized signs and symptoms, developed coping strategies, found ways to communicate your needs, and learned how to keep problems from overwhelming you again. Each bit of knowledge and practice strengthens your capacity to live more freely.

Hope does not guarantee a life without triggers or sorrow. Instead, it offers perspective: you have the tools, insight, and support to keep building a future that includes genuine connection, purpose, and, yes, joy. You can still feel fear without being ruled by it, still experience flashbacks without letting them undo all your progress, and still carry memories without letting them overshadow every bright moment.

From here on, you can continue nurturing the coping methods that serve you best and remain open to learning new ones if circumstances change. You can refine your boundaries in relationships, speak your truth honestly, and find communities that uplift rather than drain you. Through patience, acceptance, and a willingness to keep trying, you make space for hope to live beside any lingering hurt.

As you finish reading, remember: You are allowed to honor where you have been and simultaneously anticipate what lies ahead. The trauma happened, but you are more than that event—you are a person with dreams, strengths, and a unique path that can still flourish. May you go forward with renewed assurance that, although you may still carry scars, they do not bar you from embracing tomorrow. They can become part of a life story where healing, resilience, and the power of hope light the way.

Made in the USA
Coppell, TX
04 February 2025

45425195R00109